Child Advocacy in Action

Editors

LISA J. CHAMBERLAIN
TINA L. CHENG
DAVID M. KELLER

PEDIATRIC CLINICS
OF NORTH AMERICA

www.pediatric.theclinics.com

Consulting Editor
TINA L. CHENG

February 2023 • Volume 70 • Number 1

ELSEVIER

1600 John F. Kennedy Boulevard • Suite 1800 • Philadelphia, Pennsylvania, 19103-2899

http://www.theclinics.com

THE PEDIATRIC CLINICS OF NORTH AMERICA Volume 70, Number 1
February 2023 ISSN 0031-3955, ISBN-13: 978-0-323-93845-7

Editor: Kerry Holland
Developmental Editor: Axell Ivan Jade M. Purificacion

The Pediatric Clinics of North America (ISSN 0031-3955) is published bimonthly by Elsevier Inc., 360 Park Avenue South, New York, NY 10010-1710. Months of issue are February, April, June, August, October, and December. Periodicals postage paid at New York, NY and additional mailing offices. Subscription prices are $279.00 per year (US individuals), $827.00 per year (US institutions), $351.00 per year (Canadian individuals), $1100.00 per year (Canadian institutions), $419.00 per year (international individuals), $1100.00 per year (international institutions), $100.00 per year (US students and residents), $100.00 per year (Canadian students and residents), and $165.00 per year (international residents and students). To receive students/resident rare, orders must be accompanied by name of affiliated institution, date of term, and the signature of program/residency coordinator on institution letterhead. Orders will be billed at individual rate until proof of status is received. Foreign air speed delivery is included in all *Clinics* subscription prices. All prices are subject to change without notice. **POSTMASTER:** Send address changes to *The Pediatric Clinics of North America*, Elsevier Health Sciences Division, Subscription Customer Service, 3251 Riverport Lane, Maryland Heights, MO 63043. **Customer Service: 1-800-654-2452 (US and Canada). From outside of the US and Canada: 1-314-447-8871. Fax: 1-314-447-8029. For print support, E-mail: JournalsCustomerService-usa@elsevier. com. For online support, E-mail: JournalsOnlineSupport-usa@elsevier.com**.

Reprints. For copies of 100 or more, of articles in this publication, please contact the Commercial Reprints Department, Elsevier Inc., 360 Park Avenue South, New York, NY 10010-1710. Tel.: 212-633-3874; Fax: 212-633-3820; E-mail: reprints@elsevier.com.

The Pediatric Clinics of North America is also published in Spanish by McGraw-Hill Inter-americana Editores S.A., Mexico City, Mexico; in Portuguese by Riechmann and Affonso Editores, Rua Comandante Coelho 1085, CEP 21250, Rio de Janeiro, Brazil; and in Greek by Althayia SA, Athens, Greece.

The Pediatric Clinics of North America is covered in *MEDLINE/PubMed (Index Medicus), Excerpta Medica, Current Contents, Current Contents/Clinical Medicine, Science Citation Index, ASCA, ISI/BIOMED,* and *BIOSIS.*

PROGRAM OBJECTIVE

The goal of the *Pediatric Clinics of North America* is to keep practicing physicians and residents up to date with current clinical practice in pediatrics by providing timely articles reviewing the state-of-the-art in patient care.

TARGET AUDIENCE

All practicing pediatricians, physicians, and healthcare professionals who provide patient care to pediatric patients.

LEARNING OBJECTIVES

Upon completion of this activity, participants will be able to:
1. Review the levels and tiered strategy used by pediatricians to encourage child advocacy.
2. Discuss the advantages of incorporating advocacy as a skill and advocacy activities into medical education.
3. Recognize advocacy as a powerful tool used by pediatricians and healthcare team members to improve children's health and well-being.

ACCREDITATIONS

Physician Credit

The Elsevier Office of Continuing Medical Education (EOCME) is accredited by the Accreditation Council for Continuing Medical Education (ACCME) to provide continuing medical education for physicians.

The EOCME designates this journal-based activity for a maximum of 15 *AMA PRA Category 1 Credit*(s)™. Physicians should claim only the credit commensurate with the extent of their participation in the activity.

All other healthcare professionals requesting continuing education credit for this journal-based activity will be issued a certificate of participation.

ABP Maintenance of Certification Credit

Successful completion of this CME activity, which includes participation in the activity and individual assessment of and feedback to the learner, enables the learner to earn up to 15 MOC points in the American Board of Pediatrics' (ABP) Maintenance of Certification (MOC) program. It is the CME activity provider's responsibility to submit learner completion information to ACCME for the purpose of granting ABP MOC credit.

DISCLOSURE OF CONFLICTS OF INTEREST

The EOCME assesses conflict of interest with its instructors, faculty, planners, and other individuals who are in a position to control the content of CME activities. All relevant conflicts of interest that are identified are thoroughly vetted by EOCME for fair balance, scientific objectivity, and patient care recommendations. EOCME is committed to providing its learners with CME activities that promote improvements or quality in healthcare and not a specific proprietary business or a commercial interest.

The planning committee, staff, authors, and editors listed below have identified no financial relationships or relationships to products or devices they or their spouse/life partner have with commercial interest related to the content of this CME activity:
James Baumberger, MPP; Lee Savio Beers, MD; Deanna Behrens, MD; Debra L. Best, MD; Sara M. Bode, MD; Karen Camero, MD; Lisa Chamberlain, MD, MPH, FAAP; Tina L. Cheng, MD, MPH; Scott C. Denne, MD; James Dodington, MD; Maya Haasz, MD; Nia Heard-Garris, MD, MSc, FAAP; Joyce R. Javier, MD, MPH, MS, FAAP; Tiffani J. Johnson, MD, MSc; Christopher D. Kassotis, PhD; David Keller, MD, FAAP; Perri Klass, MD, FAAP; Jonathan D. Klein, MD, MPH; Lois K. Lee, MD, MPH; Keila N. Lopez, MD, MPH; Rajkumar Mayakrishnan, BSc, MBA; Dipesh Navsaria, MPH, MSLIS, MD, FAAP; Abby L. Nerlinger, MD, MPH; Lynn Olson, PhD; Christian D. Pulcini, MD, MEd, MPH; Jean L. Raphael, MD, MPH; Elissa A. Resnick, MPH; Felicia Scott-Wellington, MD; Anita N. Shah, DO, MPH; Shetal Shah, MD, FAAP; Doreen Thomas-Payne, MSN, BSN, RN, PMHNP-BC; Leonardo Trasande, MD, MPP; Melinda A. Williams-Willingham, MD, FAAP; Paul H. Wise, MD, MPH; Joseph L. Wright, MD, MPH

UNAPPROVED/OFF-LABEL USE DISCLOSURE

The EOCME requires CME faculty to disclose to the participants:
1. When products or procedures being discussed are off-label, unlabelled, experimental, and/or investigational (not US Food and Drug Administration [FDA] approved); and

2. Any limitations on the information presented, such as data that are preliminary or that represent ongoing research, interim analyses, and/or unsupported opinions. Faculty may discuss information about pharmaceutical agents that is outside of FDA-approved labelling. This information is intended solely for CME and is not intended to promote off-label use of these medications. If you have any questions, contact the medical affairs department of the manufacturer for the most recent prescribing information.

TO ENROLL

To enroll in the *Pediatric Clinics of North America* Continuing Medical Education program, call customer service at 1-800-654-2452 or sign up online at http://www.theclinics.com/home/cme. The CME program is available to subscribers for an additional annual fee of USD 324.00.

METHOD OF PARTICIPATION

In order to claim credit, participants must complete the following:
1. Complete enrolment as indicated above.
2. Read the activity.
3. Complete the CME Test and Evaluation. Participants must achieve a score of 70% on the test. All CME Tests and Evaluations must be completed online.

In order to claim MOC points, participants must complete the following:
1. Complete steps listed above for claiming CME credit
2. Provide your specialty board ID#, birth date (MM/DD), and attestation.
3. Online MOC submission is only available for the American Board of pediatrics' (ABP) Maintenance of Certification (MOC) program

CME INQUIRIES/SPECIAL NEEDS

For all CME inquiries or special needs, please contact elsevierCME@elsevier.com.

Contributors

CONSULTING EDITOR

TINA L. CHENG, MD, MPH
BK Rachford Professor and Chair of Pediatrics, University of Cincinnati, Director, Cincinnati Children's Research Foundation, Chief Medical Officer, Cincinnati Children's Hospital Medical Center, Cincinnati, Ohio

EDITORS

LISA J. CHAMBERLAIN, MD, MPH
Professor of Pediatrics, Stanford School of Medicine, Professor by Courtesy, Stanford Graduate School of Education, Arline and Pete Harman Faculty Scholar, Associate Chair, Policy and Community Engagement, Lucile Packard Children's Hospital, Stanford, California

TINA L. CHENG, MD, MPH
BK Rachford Professor and Chair of Pediatrics, University of Cincinnati, Director, Cincinnati Children's Research Foundation, Chief Medical Officer, Cincinnati Children's Hospital Medical Center, Cincinnati, Ohio

DAVID M. KELLER, MD, FAAP
Professor, University of Colorado School of Medicine, Vice Chair, Clinical Strategy and Transformation, Department of Pediatrics, Children's Hospital Colorado, Aurora, Colorado

AUTHORS

JAMES BAUMBERGER, MPP
Senior Director, Federal Advocacy, American Academy of Pediatrics, Washington, DC

LEE SAVIO BEERS, MD
Child Health Advocacy Institute, Children's National Hospital, Metro Shaw, Washington, DC

DEANNA BEHRENS, MSME, MD
Division of Pediatric Critical Care, Department of Pediatrics, Advocate Children's Hospital, Park Ridge, Illinois

DEBRA L. BEST, MD
Associate Professor, Department of Pediatrics, Duke University School of Medicine, Division of General Pediatrics and Adolescent Health, Durham, North Carolina

SARA M. BODE, MD
Associate Professor, Department of Pediatrics, Nationwide Children's Hospital, Columbus, Ohio

KAREN CAMERO, MD
General Academic Pediatrics in Health Equity Fellow, Children's Hospital Los Angeles, Los Angeles, California

LISA J. CHAMBERLAIN, MD, MPH
Professor of Pediatrics, Stanford School of Medicine, Professor by Courtesy, Stanford Graduate School of Education, Arline and Pete Harman Faculty Scholar, Associate Chair, Policy and Community Engagement, Lucile Packard Children's Hospital, Stanford, California

TINA L. CHENG, MD, MPH
BK Rachford Professor and Chair of Pediatrics, University of Cincinnati, Director, Cincinnati Children's Research Foundation, Chief Medical Officer, Cincinnati Children's Hospital Medical Center, Cincinnati, Ohio

SCOTT C. DENNE, MD
Professor of Pediatrics, Vice Chair for Clinical Research, Indiana University School of Medicine, Riley Hospital for Children, Indianapolis, Indiana

JAMES DODINGTON, MD
Section of Pediatric Emergency Medicine, Yale School of Medicine, New Haven, Connecticut

MAYA HAASZ, MD
Section of Emergency Medicine, Children's Hospital Colorado, Aurora, Colorado

NIA HEARD-GARRIS, MD, MSC, FAAP
Assistant Professor of Pediatrics, Division of Advanced General Pediatrics and Primary Care, Mary Ann & J. Milburn Smith Child Health Outreach, Research, and Evaluation Center, Ann & Robert H. Lurie Children's Hospital of Chicago, Department of Pediatrics, Northwestern University Feinberg School of Medicine, Chicago, Illinois

JOYCE R. JAVIER, MD, MPH, MS, FAAP
Associate Professor of Clinical Pediatrics, Department of Pediatrics, Division of General Pediatrics, Department of Population and Public Health Sciences, Children's Hospital Los Angeles, Keck School of Medicine of USC, Los Angeles, California

TIFFANI J. JOHNSON, MD, MSc
Department of Emergency Medicine, University of California, Davis, Sacramento, California

CHRISTOPHER D. KASSOTIS, PhD
Assistant Professor, Institute of Environmental Health Sciences, Department of Pharmacology, Wayne State University, Detroit, Michigan

DAVID M. KELLER, MD, FAAP
Professor, University of Colorado School of Medicine, Vice Chair, Clinical Strategy and Transformation, Department of Pediatrics, Children's Hospital Colorado, Aurora, Colorado

PERRI KLASS, MD, FAAP
Department of Pediatrics, Grossman School of Medicine, Arthur L. Carter Journalism Institute, New York University, New York, New York, USA

JONATHAN D. KLEIN, MD, MPH
Associate Vice Chancellor for Research, Samuel and Savithri Raj Professor, Executive Vice Head of Pediatrics, Department of Pediatrics, University of Illinois Chicago, Chicago, Illinois

LOIS K. LEE, MD, MPH
Division of Emergency Medicine, Boston Children's Hospital, Boston, Massachusetts

KEILA N. LOPEZ, MD, MPH
Department of Pediatrics, Baylor College of Medicine, Houston, Texas

DIPESH NAVSARIA, MPH, MSLIS, MD, FAAP
Associate Professor of Pediatrics and Human Development and Family Studies, School of Medicine & Public Health, School of Human Ecology, University of Wisconsin-Madison, Madison, Wisconsin

ABBY L. NERLINGER, MD, MPH
Assistant Professor, Department of Pediatrics, Duke University School of Medicine, Division of General Pediatrics and Adolescent Health, Durham, North Carolina

LYNN OLSON, PhD
Vice President of Research, American Academy of Pediatrics, Itasca, Illinois

CHRISTIAN D. PULCINI, MD, MEd, MPH
Department of Emergency Medicine and Pediatrics, University of Vermont Larner College of Medicine, Burlington, Vermont

JEAN L. RAPHAEL, MD, MPH
Department of Pediatrics, Baylor College of Medicine, Houston, Texas

ELISSA A. RESNICK, MPH
Senior Research Specialist, Department of Pediatrics, University of Illinois Chicago, Chicago, Illinois

FELICIA SCOTT-WELLINGTON, MD
Adolescent Medicine Attending Physician, Assistant Professor of Clinical Pediatrics, Department of Pediatrics, University of Illinois Chicago, Chicago, Illinois

ANITA N. SHAH, DO, MPH
Assistant Professor, Department of Pediatrics, University of Cincinnati, Division of Hospital Medicine, Cincinnati Children's Hospital Medical Center, Cincinnati, Ohio

SHETAL SHAH, MD, FAAP
Clinical Professor of Pediatrics, Division of Newborn Medicine, Department of Pediatrics, Maria Fareri Children's Hospital, New York Medical College, Valhalla, New York

LEONARDO TRASANDE, MD, MPP
Professor, Department of Pediatrics, Division of Environmental Pediatrics, Department of Population Health, Department of Environmental Medicine, NYU Grossman School of Medicine, NYU Wagner School of Public Service, NYU School of Global Public Health, New York, New York

MELINDA A. WILLIAMS-WILLINGHAM, MD
InTouch Pediatrics, Snellville, Georgia

PAUL H. WISE, MD, MPH
Richard E. Behrman Professor of Child Health and Society, Professor of Pediatrics, Senior Fellow, Freeman Spogli Institute for International Studies, Stanford University Encina Commons, Stanford, California

JOSEPH L. WRIGHT, MD, MPH
Department of Pediatrics, University of Maryland School of Medicine, Vice President and Chief Health Equity Officer, University of Maryland Medical System, Baltimore, Maryland; Department of Health Policy and Management, University of Maryland School of Public Health, College Park, Maryland

Contents

Advocacy within Healthcare

The notion that the physician has a responsibility to both the patient in their care and the community in which they reside has been a source of inspiration and tension within the profession for centuries. The profession of Pediatrics has uniquely incorporated advocacy into its training programs and will likely continue to incorporate advocacy into its professional standards for the foreseeable future. In this article, we review the history of advocacy within the profession, outline the skills needs for successful child health advocacy and offer examples of how advocacy combined with pediatric practice has improved the lives of children.

Pediatricians are effective advocates to improve the health and well-being of children, yet there are limited avenues by which to pursue academic promotion based on these activities. Drawing on an expanded definition of scholarship, pediatric advocates can use the portfolio format to highlight the quantity, quality, and impact of advocacy activities. True congruence with research and education will only be achieved through recognition and value by institutions and organizations.

Effective child health advocacy is an essential strategy to improve child health, and can improve access to equitable care. It can also be professionally rewarding and improve career satisfaction. However, while advocacy has been a part of pediatrics since its origins as a specialty, many barriers to engaging in health advocacy exist which can be challenging to navigate. There are a wide range of organizational practice settings, which are each accompanied by unique strengths and limitations. No matter the practice setting, pediatricians can be effective advocates for child health through leveraging organizational, professional, and community resources and partnerships.

Advocacy in the Community

Pediatricians play a critical role in promoting child health through community engagement, yet the skills required to be effective leaders and advocates alongside the community are often not the focus of traditional medical training. The American Academy of Pediatrics Community

women and children across racial and ethnic groups. To understand who is included in clinical research, data are required. A personal journey of advocacy requiring the National Institutes of Health to report inclusion in clinical studies by age was ultimately accomplished by federal legislation.

The last several years have seen accelerated activity and discourse directed at antiracism. Specifically following the 2020 murder of George Floyd, institutions across the country engaged in a range of introspective exercises and transparent reckonings examining their practices, policies, and history insofar as equity and racism is concerned. The authors of this article, both active protagonists in this domain, have been, and continue to be, part of ongoing national efforts and have learned much about the strategies and tactics necessary to initiate, engage, and sustain traction on the path to antiracism.

During 2021, nearly 150,000 unaccompanied children (UCs) were apprehended at the US–Mexican border. Most are leaving Guatemala, Honduras, and El Salvador, motivated by poverty, climate change, and violence. UCs are most often apprehended by the Border Patrol and then transferred to the Office of Refugee Resettlement (ORR), the Department of Health and Human Services. ORR is responsible for ensuring that the child is released to a parent or sponsor in the United States capable of providing an adequate home. Advocacy must not only address a complex system of legal and custodial care but also confront a troubled political environment.

Global Child Advocacy

Tobacco and secondhand smoke remain leading threats to public health. Evidence since the 1950s has shown that the tobacco industry has acted in bad faith to deceive the public about the health effects of smoking. They have specifically targeted vulnerable populations including children and adolescents with various—and often misleading—marketing efforts and promotions. The increased popularity and weak regulation of electronic cigarettes have created a new generation of smokers who mistakenly believe they are "safer" from harm. Continued research, advocacy, and government action are needed to protect public health. Public health advocates must know the evidence, build coalitions, and prepare for industry countermeasures. Persistence is key, but public health efforts have successfully decreased tobacco-related deaths.

Children suffer disproportionately from disease and disability due to environmental hazards, for reasons rooted in their biology. The contribution is substantial and increasingly recognized, particularly due to ever-increasing awareness of endocrine disruption. Regulatory actions can be traced directly to reductions in toxic exposures, with tangible benefits to society. Deep flaws remain in the policy framework in industrialized countries, failing to offer sufficient protection, but are even more limited in industrializing nations where the majority of chemical production and use will occur by 2030. Evidence-based steps for reducing chemical exposures associated with adverse health outcomes exist and should be incorporated into anticipatory guidance.

Advocacy to Action

Research has led to major achievements in public policy and child health. Despite the gains, the need for research to inform policy remains paramount against a backdrop of inadequate public health investments, health inequities, and public skepticism toward science. However, the translation of research into child health policy has often been slow due to misalignments in incentives between researchers and policy makers and a paucity of conceptual models to inform translation. This article outlines barriers to translation, provides examples of discordance between evidence and policy, summarizes models to inform translation, and offers strategies to improve translation of research to policy.

Clinicians who want to communicate child advocacy messages, stories, and arguments can draw on their clinical and scientific experience, but effective communication to wider—and nonmedical—audiences requires careful thought. We discuss choosing and honing the message, developing writing and speaking skills that fit both the exigencies of the chosen medium and format, including op-eds, essays, social media, public testimony, and speeches. We provide guidance on proposing articles, working with editors, shaping language and diction for a general audience, and drawing on clinical experiences while respecting confidentiality. all with the goal of effective communication, spoken and written, in the service of children and child advocacy

With greater understanding of the impact of social determinants on child health, advocacy has become essential to promoting children's health, particularly at the population level. Successful advocacy requires coalition building. Steps on how to create a productive coalition, including the selection of partner organizations, understanding how these groups enhance your activities, and strict definition of assigned roles is reviewed. Examples of successful coalitions are reviewed. A list of potential partners, who focus on various aspects of child health, is provided.

PEDIATRIC CLINICS OF NORTH AMERICA

THE CLINICS ARE AVAILABLE ONLINE!
Access your subscription at:
www.theclinics.com

Foreword

Child Advocacy in Action

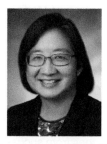

Tina L. Cheng, MD, MPH
Consulting Editor

Child health professionals are natural advocates. We recognize the great potential of each child and the importance of investing early for healthy children and the adults they will become. We see social inequities affecting child health and work to make an impact child by child, family by family, and through advocacy. Children can't vote, so we must stand and vote for them.

There is much to learn from success stories in advocacy. This issue offers case studies of child advocacy in action. It also offers tools on effective advocacy. Isaacs and Schroeder[1] reviewed major public health successes over the past decades in an article entitled "Where the public good prevailed: lessons from success stories in health." In reviewing successes, including reductions in cavities with fluoride, reducing lead poisoning, reducing traffic fatalities, and reducing smoking, they identified four ingredients of success: (1) **Highly credible scientific evidence** that persuades policymakers and withstands attack from those whose interests are threatened; (2) **Passionate advocates** who are committed and unrelenting; (3) **Partnership with the media** for public awareness and action; and (4) **Law and regulation** often at the federal level. On highly credible scientific evidence, an article in this issue discusses translating research to policy. On passionate advocates, we are the passionate advocates. Passion is illustrated in the case studies in this issue. On partnership with the media, the articles on child advocacy communication and child advocacy collaboration offer direction. Finally, law and regulation are highlighted in many of the case studies.

https://doi.org/10.1016/j.pcl.2022.10.001
0031-3955/23/© 2022 Elsevier Inc. All rights reserved.
pediatric.theclinics.com

To create change, it has been said that we need the Wisdom, the Will, and the Wallet for child advocacy.[2] We hope that this issue inspires your wisdom and will and strengthens your voice for children, adolescents, and families.

Tina L. Cheng, MD, MPH
Department of Pediatrics
University of Cincinnati College of Medicine
Cincinnati Children's Hospital Medical Center
3333 Burnet Avenue, MLC 3016
Cincinnati, OH 45229, USA

E-mail address:
Tina.Cheng@cchmc.org

REFERENCES

1. Isaacs SL, Schroeder SA. Where the public good prevailed: lessons from success stories in health, vol. 12. The American Prospect; 2001. p. 26–30.
2. Cheng TL. Academic Pediatric Association (APA) presidential address: the wisdom, the will, and the wallet: leadership on behalf of kids and families. Acad Pediatr 2010;10(2):81–6.

Advocacy within Healthcare

Child Advocacy in Action
If Not You, Who? If Not now, When?

David M. Keller, MD*

KEYWORDS

- Advocacy • Child health • Politics • State • History of pediatrics • Health policy
- Federal

KEY POINTS

- Various forms of advocacy have been part of the practice of medicine for millennia.
- Within the United States, Pediatrics formed as a specialty in part because of the need to advocate for societal responses to address the health problems of children.
- The skills of effective advocacy can be defined, practiced, and taught.

Inferior doctors treat the patient's disease; Mediocre doctors treat the patient as a person; Superior doctors treat the community as a whole.
–Huangdi Neijing, 2600 bc (apocryphal)[1]

Although translators may differ on the translation of the original Chinese, the notion that the physician has a responsibility to both the patient in their care and the community in which they reside has been a source of inspiration and tension within the profession for centuries. Hippocrates[2] and Maimonides[3] focused on the art of medicine in the oaths attributed to their names, recognizing that physicians must be careful not to abuse the powers granted to them by society in order to be effective in the diagnosis and treatment of disease. The obligation to the patient was clear, and it could be inferred that one should advocate on behalf of that patient to assure access to the medications, facilities, and procedures that would help to restore the patient's health. As the science of Western medicine developed in nineteenth century Europe, the role of the physician changed.[4] Although some physicians embraced a science-based model focused on the individual,[5] others realized health was the result of several factors, many of which were environmental and societal. Famously, in 1854, John Snow

ª Department of Pediatrics, Clinical Strategy & Transformation, University of Colorado, School of Medicine, Children's Hospital Colorado, 13123 East 16th Avenue, Box 065, Aurora, CO 80045, USA; ᵇ Stanford School of Medicine, Stanford Graduate School of Education, Policy & Community Engagement; ᶜ University of Cincinnati, Cincinnati Children's Research Foundation, Cincinnati Children's Hospital Medical Center, 3333 Burnet Avenue MLC 3016, Cincinnati, OH 45229-3026, USA
* Corresponding author.
E-mail address: David.keller@childrenscolorado.org

Pediatr Clin N Am 70 (2023) 1–10
https://doi.org/10.1016/j.pcl.2022.09.004
0031-3955/23/© 2022 Elsevier Inc. All rights reserved.

recognized the foul water of the Broad St pump as the source of cholera in London, taking action to stop the epidemic at its source rather than at the bedside.[6] A few years earlier in 1848, Rudolf Virchow had seen the relationship between poverty and disease in his seminal study *"Report on the Typhus Epidemic in Upper Silesia,"* creating the foundations of public health and social medicine.[7] Virchow's observation that "Medicine is a social science and politics is nothing else but medicine on a large scale" has long served as a call to physicians to engage in advocacy for a healthier society, leading to physician engagement at the community and political levels.[8] Some have argued that such engagement would diminish our effectiveness as healers, reducing public trust and interfering with our ability to care for the individuals who present for care.[9,10] Others hold that this is central to our work and should be a foundational pillar of our profession.[11–13] This is especially true in Pediatrics, a specialty that, one could argue, developed from the realization that child health is inextricably bound to the social and environmental milieu in which the child is raised.

Often cited as the father of pediatrics, Abraham Jacobi was, as noted in a 1997 article by Robert Haggerty, a "respectable rebel."[14] Born and educated in Germany, he immigrated to the United States after being imprisoned for associating with radicals during the uprisings of 1848 and established a practice in Manhattan among the immigrant population.[15] By 1860, he had written the first pediatric textbook in America, "Midwifery and Diseases of Women and Children," and was appointed Professor of Pediatrics at New York Medical College. He was an extraordinary clinician, teacher, and researcher, publishing more than 8 volumes of research during his lifetime. Most notably, however, he was an advocate. At the founding of the American Pediatric Society (APS) in 1886, he wrote "Questions of public hygiene and medicine are both professional and social. Thus, every physician is by destiny a citizen of the commonwealth with many rights and great responsibilities."[16] The professional commitment of pediatricians to advocacy has continued over the century and a half since Jacobi's time.

Jacobi was one of many new immigrants who came to the United States at the end of the nineteenth century. Many others were not as successful in adapting to American society. In the early nineteenth century, with increasing income inequality and urban industrialization, it was clear that the health of the population was tied closely to the social environment in which the population was living. Leaders such as Jane Addams of Hull House in Chicago developed novel programs, including kindergarten and nurseries, to support poor families as they tried to maintain their families in spite of the harsh conditions.[17] Ms. Addams also worked with her colleagues, Julia Lathrop and Lucy Flowers, to change the ways in which children were handled in the juvenile justice system. The efforts of these leaders and others in the Progressive movement led to the first White House Conference on the Care of Dependent Children in 1909, bringing the Federal government into the discussion and informing the child health advocacy agenda for decades to come.[18]

Amid the tumult of the Progressive Era, Pediatrics continued to evolve as a profession.[19] Julia Lathrop established the Children's Bureau in 1912 and created a nationwide plan to reduce maternal and child mortality that formed the basis of the Sheppard-Towner Act of 1921.[20] Although the Pediatric Section of the American Medical Association (AMA) supported the maternal and child health interventions initiated under the Sheppard-Towner act, most of organized medicine opposed what was described as a socialist intervention, ultimately leading to the formation of the American Academy of Pediatrics (AAP) as an independent body.[21] Pediatricians such as Julius Richmond were instrumental in the establishment of Medicare, Medicaid, and Headstart during the 1960s, leading to tremendous improvements in access to health care as well as child health and development.[22] The APS, along with newer organizations including the Ambulatory (now Academic) Pediatric Association (APA), the Society for Pediatric Research (SPR), and the Association of Medical School Pediatric Department Chairs (AMSPDC) have formed the Pediatric Policy Council to work with the AAP to ensure that the voice of children is heard within the halls of government.[23]

The AAP also established the Community Access to Child Health (CATCH) program as a way to support its members who wished to engage in partnership with community organizations to address child health issues in their own communities.[16] Ultimately, this led to the incorporation of advocacy into the Pediatric Residency program require-ments. Since 1996, in order to become a pediatrician, "there must be structured educational experiences that prepare residents for the role of advocate for the health of children within the community."[24] That requirement has been modified several times but remains a core component of Pediatric residency training. Finally, in a recent survey of pediatric department chairs from around the country, advocacy for child health was seen as an increasingly important part of the academic mission.[25] To quote one of the Chairs surveyed: "It is a time of increased advocacy for many areas in the society that affect child well-being. As health leaders it is our obligation to step it up." Another Chair added: "We consider advocacy as the fourth leg of the academic stool." The profession of Pediatrics began with advocacy, has uniquely incorporated advo-cacy into its training programs, and will likely continue to incorporate advocacy into its professional standards for the foreseeable future.

Exactly what is meant by advocacy in pediatrics has been discussed and refined many times over the years. Few would disagree that physicians have a duty to their patients, to "benefit my patients according to my greatest ability and judgment, and I...do no harm or injustice to them," as the Hippocratic Oath is often translated.[2] Within a hospital system, this may mean working to get one's patient quicker access to a specialized service or medication, or even transferring a patient to another's care, if necessary. Over the years, many within Pediatrics have taken a broader view, building on Dr Jacobi's vision of the unique role of physicians in the body politic. This some-times took on a paternalistic tone. Regarding the reforms of the early twentieth cen-tury, one APS leader commented "We physicians, however, whose mission it really is to guide the progress of the various reforms connected with early life and see that they do not go astray, should interest ourselves in curbing exaggerated ideas and in the prevention of unwisely pressing on our legislators unsound views on which to base new laws."[26] By the 1960s, many pediatricians had come to see community engagement as the key to improving child health, based on Philip Porter's work with the city of Cambridge, Massachusetts, and believed that pediatricians should be part of broad-based community coalitions and lead by:

1. generating creative and resourceful ideas (*knowledge base*) to address an impor-tant community need or problem;
2. giving shape and form to those ideas by developing a *social strategy* that would incorporate the most successful approaches to accomplishing a goal; and
3. marshaling the *political will* among colleagues and other community leaders to address child health issues."[16]

This approach formed the basis of the AAPs engagement in CATCH and other com-munity pediatrics initiatives for many years. In the 1990s, as advocacy training curricula were being developed, AAP President Stephen Berman called for more engagement in the legislative process by pediatricians and proposed the incorpora-tion of advocacy into the normal path of a pediatric career.[27] In the early twenty-first century, the Ambulatory Pediatric Association convened a group of "advocacy experts" to develop a consensus definition of advocacy using a modified Delphi process, in order to better focus curricular development:

"To speak up, to plead, or to champion for a cause while applying professional expertise and leadership to support efforts on individual (patient or family), community, and legislative/policy levels, which result in the improved quality of life for individuals, families, or communities."[28]

At the same time, Anne Dyson, a pediatrician and philanthropist funded the Community Pediatrics Training Initiative, later incorporated into the AAP. They developed a definition of advocacy that incorporated many similar ideas:

"Child advocacy pediatricians should advocate for the well-being of patients, families, and communities; must develop advocacy skills to address relevant individual, community, and population health issues; and understand the legislative process (local, state, and federal) to address community and child health issues."[29]

More recently, a simpler definition has been offered by Earnest and colleagues:

"Physician advocacy is action by a physician to promote those social, economic, educational, and political changes that ameliorate the suffering and threats to human health and well-being."[11]

One could simplify the definition even further, as was done by the simple assertion on Twitter by a group of Emergency Medicine physicians in the wake of mass shootings of children: #ThisIsOurLane[30]! Advocacy, however defined, has become as an essential part of pediatric training and practice, and it is becoming a larger part of the practice of medicine throughout the United States.

Despite this rich history, the Pediatric literature, like most of the medical literature, has focused on what most would view as the traditional content of academic medicine: our clinical insights, the research that moves the field forward, and the ways in which we can train the next generation of pediatric clinicians. In this volume, our goal is to provide practical advice and capture advocacy stories that have enriched our profession over the years for the pediatric advocates of the future. Similar to everything else, in Pediatrics, effective advocacy requires the development of specific skills. Although medical school and residency training can introduce these skills, they must be revisited and honed over the course of one's career in Pediatrics. Several have tried to describe the skills needs to practice advocacy as a pediatric clinician. Four examples are listed in **Table 1** within this article.

All those who advocate for advocacy point out that most advocacy is driven by one's passion within the profession, whether that be a passion for children with disabilities, families disrupted by poverty or lives lost to firearms. The passion is clear in the many case studies you will see throughout this volume. Passion allows one to focus one's energy over time, as advocacy work is not, in general, a short-term exercise. Although most of the authors highlight the unique expertise pediatric clinicians bring to an issue, all are careful to highlight the importance of networking, coalition building, and multidisciplinary teams in effective advocacy work. Dr Berman put it quite succinctly: "No one can be an advocate by themselves. You need to build and develop networks with people, organizations, coalitions."[27] Pediatric clinicians bring expertise and professionalism to any group of advocates but knowledge alone is insufficient to drive change. An understanding of systems, and where knowledge can be applied, is critical. All recognize the importance of communication in this study; many call out the importance of traditional media such as newspapers, radio, and television in articles from more than 20 years ago. To that we must add the powerful new tool of social media—Facebook, Twitter, and Instagram, which have completely changed the communication landscape. Finally, all emphasize the importance of the long view. We know this within our study with patients and families under our care.

Table 1
Skills required for effective child health advocacy

Hoffman et al[35]	Dyson Initiative[29]	Berman[27]	APA Delphi Process[28]
1. Identify and discuss individual, family, and community (local, state, and/or national) concerns that affect children's health	A. Delivery of culturally effective care: Pediatricians must demonstrate interpersonal and communication skills that result in effective information exchange with children and families from all cultural backgrounds and diverse communities	Develop a clear mission	Patient-level advocacy • Assess patient's and family's assets and needs • Screen for issues that affect child health (food, education, housing, safety) • Work collaboratively with patients, families, and community agencies
2. Formulate an attainable plan of action in response to a community health need	B. Child advocacy: Child advocacy pediatricians should advocate for the well-being of patients, families, and communities; must develop advocacy skills to address relevant individual, community, and population health issues; and understand the legislative process (local, state, and federal) to address community and child health issues	Implement a strategy of small wins	• Involve patients in decision-making • Identify appropriate local resources and steer patients toward them • Communicate effectively with patients, families, and others
3. Identify and describe resources to effectively advocate for the well-being of patients, families, and communities	C. Medical home: Pediatricians must be able to identify and/or provide a medical home for all children and families under their care	Identify friends and build coalitions	Community-level advocacy • Access community resources • Reach out on behalf of patients to other components of the health system and to public and private agencies
4. Communicate effectively with community groups and the media	D. Special populations: Pediatricians, in concert with other child health professionals, must collaboratively develop and implement management plans that are	Identify adversaries and attempt to neutralize their opposition	• Plan actions necessary to bring about desired change or results—Develop relationships with those in need in the community

(continued on next page)

Table 1
(continued)

Hoffman et al[35]	Dyson Initiative[29]	Berman[27]	APA Delphi Process[28]
realistic, family-centered, community referenced, nonrestrictive, and effective			• Work cooperatively in multidisciplinary teams
5. Find and use evidence and data to communicate, educate, effect attitude change, and/or obtain funding to achieve specific health outcomes	E. The pediatrician as a consultant, partner, and collaborative leader: Pediatricians must be able to act as child health consultants in their communities	Be pragmatic and willing to compromise	Legislative/policy advocacy • Participate in ongoing advocacy efforts within the hospital, professional groups (eg, AAP), or grass-roots efforts
6. Describe and discuss key features of the legislative process, and identify and communicate with key legislators, community leaders, child advocates, and/or agency administrators about child and family health concerns	F. Educational and childcare settings: Pediatricians must be able to interact with the staff of schools and childcare settings to improve the health and educational environments for children	Do not burn bridges and never compromise a legislator	• Describe the issues to others in understandable language and express personal experience and data with feeling • Work and collaborate with others
	G. Community and public health: Pediatricians must be able to understand and potentially modify the health determinants affecting patients and families in the community that they serve	Hire an effective lobbyist	• Incorporate scientific information in a meaningful way into documents/testimony
	H. Research and scholarship: Pediatricians should be capable of pursuing inquiries that advance the health of children, families, and communities	Develop a good working relationship with the media (newspaper, radio, and television)	
		To the extent possible, minimize looking self-serving	

It turns out to be equally true for large systems. Relationships must be built over time and the advocates writing in this volume have all devoted much time throughout their career to address the problems for which they feel the passion for change.

One of the challenges for those who engage in advocacy is determining the success of their efforts and deciding when it would be most advantageous to press the issue about which they care so passionately. Does one measure success by the relationships built, the coalitions organized, the press releases issued, the legislation passed, or the lives impacted by one's efforts? Some of these are easily quantified but the most important outcome of child health advocacy work is the one that is hardest to measure: how ready are you and your team to move your agenda when the time is right (**Box 1**)?

Work in advocacy that creates successful health policy change is seldom linear, and it is therefore difficult to capture in a simple flow diagram. Successful advocacy involves deep understanding of what makes a good policy, how that policy interacts with the political landscape at multiple levels, and the procedural path necessary to guide that policy into implementation. This process can be summarized in **Fig. 1** below, which divides the process into political and technical aspects. Although it seems that there is a line between issues, agendas, and decisions that go into the political process and the 5 components of the technical process, it is a dotted line. In reality, all 8 of these processes interact as a policy change moves through the system. The pediatric advocate must be cognizant of the processes and have the skills to manage those connections to keep the process moving forward. The authors presented in this volume have all managed that dance successfully. Their stories will aid you in your journey going forward.

Much consideration must be given to the ways advocacy can be supported over the course of a pediatric career. Professional organizations should be the first place one looks to support advocacy work. The AAP, APS, SPR, AMSPDC, AMA, and APA all have advocacy committees, as do many subspecialty societies. The AAP and the AMA have state chapters focusing on state-level advocacy issues. All support their members in advocacy work, through training, resources, and connections. Employers, both large and small, are increasingly willing to support advocacy efforts though paid

---

Box 1
Advocacy Work is Never Done

In Colorado, the AAP chapter worked for several years with the American Association of Child and Adolescent Psychiatry (AACAP) chapter and a broad coalition of other stakeholders to establish a Pediatric Mental Health Care Access program, using funding from the Health Services Resources Administration as well as the University of Colorado School of Medicine and Medicaid.[32,33] The program grew rapidly and was widely viewed by primary care physicians and families as a rousing success. The stakeholders had frequent discussions regarding sustainability of the project but had no concrete plan for funding the program when the grant expired in 2023. In 2021, when the State government decided to devote US$450M of America's Rescue Plan funding to issues of mental health, that group quickly pivoted to discussion with legislators and the governor's office regarding the success of the current program and how funding for the sustainability and expansion of the program would be a prudent use of America's Rescue Plan Act of 2021 (ARPA) dollars. Their efforts resulted in legislation that passed almost unanimously, supporting that program going forward for an additional 3 years.[34] A huge success, based on years of preparation, a strong coalition and, frankly, a bit of luck. The journey, however, is not completed. The program needs to be implemented, integrated with other parts of a rapidly changing mental health system and sustained into the future. In Colorado, after a brief celebration, the AAP and AACAP are already moving on the next stages of the journey. Although they can count a success, the study is hardly over, a sentiment with which the authors in this volume would likely agree.

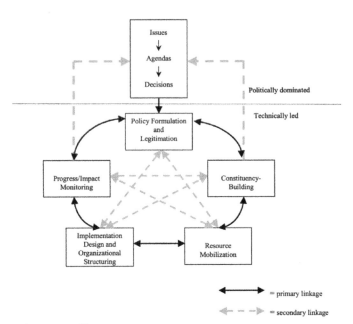

Fig. 1. The policy process[36]

leave, fundraising, or other means. Finally, academic institutions are starting to recognize advocacy as a potential vehicle for scholarly endeavors that can support career advancement for junior faculty. Whether working in the public sector, within academe or in private practice, pediatricians with the passion for change have been able to support their advocacy work in real life.

The articles in this volume should be seen as a survey of the field of advocacy within pediatrics, looking at advocacy at the community, state, federal, and global levels on a variety of issues. We have requested the authors to include real-life examples of how advocacy works, illustrating many of the skills cited above. We have also included special articles on some of the structural supports needed for effective advocacy, such as how research can inform advocacy, how one can develop the kind of networks needed for effective advocacy, and how we can write to show not just our expertise, but our passion as well. This volume is by no means comprehensive but we believe that it will be helpful to those who want to know how they can incorporate this study into their professional lives and inspire action. There is so much work to do. In the end, as former APA President Peter Szilagyi emphasized through his term of office, "It's all about the children."[31]

CLINICS CARE POINTS

- Advocacy is an essential skill in the care of children and families, with a long tradition in the practice of pediatrics.
- Child health providers should be mindful in choosing the level of advocacy in which they choose to engage (individual, local, or national) because the effort can be as overwhelming as it is rewarding.
- Advocacy is a team sport; by building the right team, pediatricians are more likely to be successful and to have fun doing it.

DISCLOSURE

The authors confirm that that they have no conflicts of interest to disclose in the preparation of this article.

REFERENCES

1. Veith I. The Yellow Emperor's Classic of Internal Medicine. New edition. Berkeley (CA): University of California Press; 1972. p. 296. ISBN 10 0520288262.
2. North Mt. Hippocratic Oath. National Library of Medicine. 2022. Available at: https://www.nlm.nih.gov/hmd/greek/greek_oath.html.
3. Prayer of maimonides. Cal State J Med 1918;16(1):1.
4. Brosco JP. Navigating the future through the past: the enduring historical legacy of federal children's health programs in the United States. Am J Public Health 2012;102(10):1848–57.
5. Pearson HA. Centennial history of the APS. Pediatr Res 1990;27(6 Suppl):S4–7.
6. Tulchinsky TH. John Snow, Cholera, the Broad Street Pump; Waterborne Diseases Then and Now. Case Stud Public Health 2018;77–99. https://doi.org/10.1016/B978-0-12-804571-8.00017-2.
7. Virchow R. Report on the Typhus Epidemic in Upper Silesia. Am J Public Health 2006;96(12):4.
8. Mackenbach JP. Politics is nothing but medicine at a larger scale: reflections on public health's biggest idea. *J Epidemiol Community Health* Mar 2009;63(3): 181–4. https://doi.org/10.1136/jech.2008.077032.
9. Huddle TS. Perspective: Medical professionalism and medical education should not involve commitments to political advocacy. *Acad Med* Mar 2011;86(3): 378–83. https://doi.org/10.1097/ACM.0b013e3182086efe.
10. Kanter SL. On physician advocacy. *Acad Med* Sep 2011;86(9):1059–60. https://doi.org/10.1097/ACM.0b013e318227744d.
11. Earnest MA, Wong SL, Federico SG. Perspective: Physician advocacy: what is it and how do we do it? Acad Med 2010;85(1):63–7. https://doi.org/10.1097/ACM.0b013e3181c40d40.
12. Sklar DP. Why Effective Health Advocacy Is So Important Today. Acad Med 2016; 91(10):1325–8. https://doi.org/10.1097/ACM.0000000000001338.
13. Shah SI, Brumberg HL. Advocating for advocacy in pediatrics: supporting life-long career trajectories. Pediatrics 2014;134(6):e1523–7. https://doi.org/10.1542/peds.2014-0211.
14. Haggerty RJ. Abraham Jacobi, MD, respectable rebel. Pediatrics 1997;99(3): 462–6. https://doi.org/10.1542/peds.99.3.462.
15. Burke EC. Abraham Jacobi, MD: the man and his legacy. Pediatrics 1998;101(2): 309–12. https://doi.org/10.1542/peds.101.2.309.
16. Hutchins VL, Grason H, Aliza B, et al. Community Access to Child Health (CATCH) in the historical context of Community Pediatrics. Pediatr 1999;103(6 Pt 3):1373–83.
17. Jane Addams DIgital project. 2022. https://digital.janeaddams.ramapo.edu/about/.
18. The story of the white House conferences on children and youth. 1967. https://eric.ed.gov/?id=ED078896.
19. Centennial Series. The Progressive Movement. Children's Bur Express 2011; 12(8):2.
20. Children's Bureau USDoHHS. The Children's Bureau legacy: ensuring the right to childhood. Washington, DC: U.S. Government Printing Office; 2012. p. 233.

21. Baker J. Women and the Invention of Well Child Care. Pediatrics 1994;94(4):5.
22. Winickoff JP, Perrin JM. A tribute to Julius B. Richmond, MD. Ambul Pediatr 2008; 8(6):349–50. https://doi.org/10.1016/j.acap.2008.10.003.
23. Block RWDB, Alan R, Cohen AR, et al. An Agenda for Children for the 113th Congress: Recommendations From the Pediatric Academic Societies. Pediatrics 2012;131(1):11.
24. ACGME. Program Requirements for residency education in pediatrics. 1996.
25. Chung RJ, Ramirez MR, Best DL, et al. Advocacy and Community Engagement: Perspectives from Pediatric Department Chairs. J Pediatr 2022. https://doi.org/10.1016/j.jpeds.2021.12.019.
26. TM R. The position and work of the American Pediatric Society toward public question. Trans Am Pediatr Soc 1909;21:8.
27. Berman S. Training Pediatricians to Become Child Advocates. Pediatrics 1998; 102(3):5.
28. Wright CJ, Katcher ML, Blatt SD, et al. Toward the development of advocacy training curricula for pediatric residents: a national delphi study. Ambul Pediatr May-Jun 2005;5(3):165–71. https://doi.org/10.1367/A04-113R.1.
29. Rezet B, Risko W, Blaschke GS. Dyson Community Pediatrics Training Initiative Curriculum C. Competency in community pediatrics: consensus statement of the Dyson Initiative Curriculum Committee. Pediatrics 2005;115(4 Suppl): 1172–83. https://doi.org/10.1542/peds.2004-2825O.
30. Ranney ML, Betz ME, Dark C. #ThisIsOurLane - Firearm Safety as Health Care's Highway. N Engl J Med 2019;380(5):405–7. https://doi.org/10.1056/NEJMp1815462.
31. Szilagyi PG. Academic Pediatric Association (APA) presidential address: changing the world for children. Ambul Pediatr Sep-Oct 2008;8(5):273–8. https://doi.org/10.1016/j.ambp.2008.07.005.
32. Sullivan K, George P, Horowitz K. Addressing National Workforce Shortages by Funding Child Psychiatry Access Programs. Pediatrics 2021;147(1). https://doi.org/10.1542/peds.2019-4012.
33. Keller D, Sarvet B. Is there a psychiatrist in the house? Integrating child psychiatry into the pediatric medical home. J Am Acad Child Adolesc Psychiatry 2013; 52(1):3–5. https://doi.org/10.1016/j.jaac.2012.10.010.
34. Behavioral Health-care Services For Children: Concerning behavioral health-care integration services for children, and, in connection therewith, making an appropriation., SB22-147, Colorado General Assembly, 2022 Regular Session sess (C K 2022). 5/17/2022. Available at: https://leg.colorado.gov/bills/sb22-147. Accessed 28 June 2022.
35. Hoffman BD, Barnes M, Ferrell C, et al. The Community Health and Advocacy Milestones Profile: A Novel Tool Linking Community Pediatrics and Advocacy Training to Assessment of Milestones-Based Competence in Pediatric Residency Training. Acad Pediatr 2016;16(4):309–13. https://doi.org/10.1016/j.acap.2016.03.006.
36. Schribner SB, DW, O'Hanlon B. Policy toolkit for strengthening health sector reform. 2000. 181. 2000. Available at: https://www.hfgproject.org/policy-toolkit-strengthening-health-sector-reform-september-2000/.

Advocacy in Pediatric Academia
Charting a Path Forward

Abby L. Nerlinger, MD, MPH[a],*, Debra L. Best, MD[a],
Anita N. Shah, DO, MPH[b,c]

KEYWORDS

• Advocacy • Scholarship • Academic promotion • Community health

KEY POINTS

- Pediatricians are effective advocates to improve the health and well-being of children and communities.
- Advocacy supports institutional missions related to community health, engagement, and equity.
- There is increased demand for integration of advocacy into the academic promotions process using an expanded definition of scholarship that focuses on process rather than product.
- Academic advocates can create Advocacy Portfolios to support academic promotion, dedication of resources such as time and funding for advocacy activities, or application for advocacy-related positions.
- Full integration of advocacy into academic institutions requires advocacy activities to be valued as congruent to research, medical education, and clinical care.

INTRODUCTION

Advocacy on behalf of both patients and populations has long been considered a core tenet of pediatric physician responsibilities.[1,2] The American Academy of Pediatrics (AAP), the major professional organization dedicated to improving the health of children, was borne out of philosophic divides within the American Medical Association regarding endorsement of legislation to create centers for maternal and child health.[2] Our roots and our professional organizations have long understood the obligation of advocacy on behalf of children, yet there remains

[a] Department of Pediatrics, Division of General Pediatrics and Adolescent Health, Duke University School of Medicine, 234 Crooked Creek Parkway, Suite 110, Durham, NC 27713, USA; [b] Department of Pediatrics, University of Cincinnatie; [c] Division of Hospital Medicine, Cincinnati Children's Hospital Medical Center, 3333 Burnet Ave, MLC 9016, Cincinnati, OH 45229, USA
* Corresponding author.
E-mail address: abby.nerlinger@nemours.org

Pediatr Clin N Am 70 (2023) 11–24
https://doi.org/10.1016/j.pcl.2022.09.001
0031-3955/23/© 2022 Elsevier Inc. All rights reserved.

a disconnect surrounding how such influential work is valued by academic institutions.

The traditional scholarly roles of physician faculty at academic medical centers include that of clinical care, scholarship (classically, research), and education/teaching.[3,4] These three scholarly domains, analogous to "three legs on a stool," are viewed as critical to the mission of academic medical institutions to (1) improve the health of patients and populations; (2) provide a mechanism for scientific inquiry that continues to advance clinical care; and (3) train the next generation. Scholarly productivity is expected of academic physicians, with the requirement to show evidence of peer review and national recognition in respective scholarly areas of focus to ascend the ladder of promotion and tenure. However, such a narrow definition of scholarship has limited recognition of achievement in domains outside of research, including advocacy.[5]

Details surrounding how advocacy fits into current academic medical institutional frameworks are an emerging area of paradigm shift that reorients institutional values around the community.[6] We argue that advocacy can be held to the same rigorous documentation and evaluation standards as traditional scholarship through the use of an Advocacy Portfolio (AP) during the academic promotion process. Advocacy drives academic institutional missions to a sufficient extent that it should be an independent "fourth leg" supporting the stool.

The logic model in **Fig. 1** displays key inputs and outcomes leading to the acceptance of advocacy as a scholarly endeavor. Although we acknowledge that such a paradigm shift will take decades, simultaneous bottom-up and top-down approaches are essential to continue charting a path forward for advocacy in academia.[7] From the top-down, support from academic leadership and institutions is necessary but not sufficient. The increasing use of APs by trainees and faculty will increase demand for recognition in the promotions process. It is critically important to promote a paradigm shift that recognizes advocacy as its own unique scholarly effort as it benefits our profession and ultimately our patients.

Overarching Goal: Advocacy is an academic pillar that is recognized and valued as a scholarly pursuit for academic pediatricians			
Inputs	**Outcomes**		**Impact**
Strategies	**Short-Term** (1–2 y)	**Medium-Term** (3–5 y)	**Long-Term** (5+ years)
Advocacy Portfolio publications	AAP CPTI[1] Template metrics	• Advocacy Products accepted in CV • Central repository for Advocacy Portfolios & Advocacy Projects	Accepted overarching goal Advocacy Portfolio widely accepted
Program Chair Stakeholder Engagement	AMSPDC buy in, Survey of acceptability of advocacy amongst program chairs	American Board of Pediatrics Support	Additional peer-reviewed outlets that recognize advocacy work and products
Expert Consensus on advocacy metrics, outcomes, & evaluation	Delphi method to begin evaluation of advocacy work	Consensus metrics on advocacy evaluation	Population health improvements
Education & Training Skill Development (Trainees, Faculty)	Academic Pediatric Association launch of Health Policy Scholars Program (HPSP); MOCA[2], CPTI[1]	Increased faculty development and training and established network of advocates	Physician satisfaction/joy in work/reduced burnout Evolution of the science of advocacy

[1]CPTI, Community Pediatrics Training Initiatives
[2]MOCA, Maintenance of Certification Assessment

Fig. 1. Logic model with inputs necessary to establish advocacy as a widely accepted and valued scholarly pursuit for pediatrician-advocates, and resultant outcomes and impact.

The Growing Role of Advocacy in Pediatrics

Pediatricians have persistently demonstrated dedication to advocate on behalf of patients and populations. A 2004 survey of pediatricians showed that $\geq$97% rated community participation and collective advocacy as important.[8] Subjectively, we see examples of grassroots physician advocates leveraging their influence in such domains as community engagement, media interactions, federal administrative rulemaking comment, and legislative advocacy. Highlighted examples include that of Dr Mona Hanna-Attisha using a press conference to inform the public and policymakers around the Flint lead crisis,[9,10] and Dr Colleen Kraft providing written opposition to the Department of Homeland Security policies separating immigrant children from their parents at the southwest US border.[11,12] The election of pediatrician, Dr Kim Schrier, to Congress, along with many more pediatric physicians running for state and federal seats with a focus on child health, demonstrate increasing civic engagement among pediatricians.[5,13]

Advocacy is at the core of pediatric values and additionally highlighted by its inclusion in education and training curricula.[7,14] Active engagement of trainees and junior faculty in Accreditation Council for Graduate Medical Education (ACGME) required advocacy activities, the AAP Section on Pediatric Trainees yearly Advocacy Campaign, and the newly established Academic Pediatric Association (APA) Health Policy Scholars Program are examples of the growing demand for advocacy training opportunities. A 2019 survey of 240 US medical students showed that 80% planned to become involved in health care policy issues as a physician, and greater than 60% planned to take leadership roles in such.[15]

Pediatric professional organizations have also seen an increase in advocacy activities, including training and engagement opportunities through the AAP, APA, American Pediatric Society, and the joint Pediatric Policy Council. An increasing number of pediatricians (>400 in the past 2 years) have been involved with the annual AAP Legislative Conference (email communication, May 2022), participating in legislative advocacy surrounding such topics as gun safety.

From an institutional perspective, the SARS-CoV-2 pandemic has motivated academic medical centers to improve health equity by conducting advocacy on behalf of communities.[16] Community engagement and partnerships are key to ameliorating health disparities rooted in structural racism, implicit and explicit bias, and historical mistrust, all of which have been compounded by the pandemic. This, in addition to the recent killing of George Floyd while in police custody, has highlighted the need for stronger institutional actions to address justice, equity, diversity, and inclusion.[17,18] Such initiatives have strengthened institutional commitments to the recruitment of faculty that reflects the diversity of patient populations served.[17] Recognition of diverse faculty experience and expertise, such as equity initiatives as a scholarly endeavor, supports the mission, vision, and values of academic institutions surrounding equity and diversity.[17]

Despite the growing role of advocacy for pediatricians, trainees, institutions, and organizations, constraints in the academic promotion process, among other factors, have limited the pursuit of advocacy as a professional endeavor.[7,19]

Historical Context: Advocacy as Scholarship

Previous investigators have acknowledged the debate surrounding advocacy on behalf of individuals versus populations as a professional obligation, in addition to its role in academic institutions.[20–22] At times, advocacy has been equated with service to the community, oftentimes expected in university settings. The increased institutional focus on original research and publishing that arose in the 1950s coincided with a decline in public engagement by academic institutions in the United States; a shift that was paralleled by a decline in the value of service as scholarship.[6] Service became less a function of public citizenship that it had been in the late 1800s through early 1900s and more a function of institutional citizenship, which was less aligned with the goals of population advocacy.

The advent of an expanded definition of scholarship proposed by Boyer has reframed the debate regarding scholarship across a range of disciplines,[23] including teaching, public health, clinical practice, quality improvement, and advocacy. This new definition was guided by surveys of attitudes and values of over 5000 faculty members at many different types of institutions of higher learning conducted by the Carnegie Foundation for the Advancement of Teaching.[23] Defining scholarship in four "separate yet overlapping" functions of *discovery, integration, application, and teaching* opened the door for academicians to be recognized not only for research but also for work in a variety of disciplines that was believed to be more reflective of both day-to-day faculty activities and community needs:[6]

What we need, then, in higher education is a reward system that reflects the diversity of our institutions and the breadth of scholarship, as well. The challenge is to strike a balance among teaching, research, and service, a position supported by two-thirds of today's faculty who conclude that, "at my institution, we need better ways, besides publication, to evaluate scholarly performance of faculty."[24]

Through the national surveys of granting agencies and journal editors conducted by Carnegie, Glassick and colleagues developed and presented consensus regarding standards of quality scholarship regardless of field of study. These standards include *clear goals, adequate preparation, appropriate methods, outstanding results, effective communication,* and *reflective critique*.[25] Faculty across the nation coalesced in the 1990s to 2010s to define scholarly standards for the evaluation of teaching.[23] In medical education, a standardized format was proposed for Educator Portfolios,[26,27] with resultant consensus on the development of an evaluation tool to measure scholarly teaching as scholarship for the purposes of promotion and tenure.[28-32] In contrast to curriculum vitae (CVs), it was determined that the portfolio format more appropriately described the career trajectory of medical educators and allowed for quantification and qualification of scholarly products outside of the traditional currency of grants and peer-reviewed publications.[25]

The last 10 years have seen a similar trajectory for advocacy in medical academia (**Fig. 2**). Certainly, organizations such as the Association of American Medical Colleges and the ACGME that create curricular frameworks and evaluation standards for trainees have had a role in pushing advocacy into academia during this time.[7,14] Dobson and colleagues surveyed 10 expert advocates to identify abilities of physician advocates. They include seeing the "bigger picture," communication, persuasion, leveraging social position, putting ideas into action, using evidence, working in teams, and working in the community.[33] The investigators note that many of the skills embodied by successful physician advocates are not captured in competencies for medical training.[33]

During the initial years of Boyer's definition of scholarship, there were many writers who expanded on the *scholarship of engagement* (or integration),[34,35] highlighting the faculty role of service to institutions and the role of institutions in civic engagement.[36] This led to an expansion of the role of the scholarship of engagement within institutions of higher learning. Interestingly, this effect was not translated broadly in schools of medicine. Although advocacy activities meet the definition of scholarship of engagement, Nerlinger and Shah have previously highlighted opportunities and

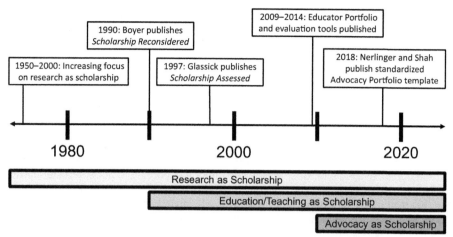

Fig. 2. The evolution of scholarship at academic medical centers, 1980-present.

challenges to applying the Glassick standards of quality scholarship to advocacy.[22] For example, the measurement of advocacy outcomes can be quite challenging due to political context, the length of time it may take to affect change, and political will.[22] These challenges highlight how fitting advocacy into tradition is akin to fitting a square peg in a round hole, the approach to which has truly limited the growth of advocacy scholarship.

Thus, academic advocates have created demand for a tool to describe the advocacy journey in a way that at CV cannot. The first standardized version of an AP was outlined by Nerlinger and Shah in 2018 in *Academic Medicine*.[22] Through expert consensus, a subsequent version has been published for electronic download through the AAP Community Pediatrics Training Initiative (AAP CPTI) Web site[37] that attempts to display the quantity, quality, and impact of scholarly advocacy work.[38]

Traditional academic pathways and the use of supporting CVs have left gaps for academic advocates. The manner with which an advocate describes their academic journey during promotion largely depends on institutional recognition, with approaches varying from turning advocacy into traditional scholarship to conducting advocacy work in a scholarly manner.[38] Each of these approaches aligns with different strategies when undergoing the promotions process. For example, some advocates will include advocacy as a separate section on the CV to align with the traditional academic pillars; others may attempt modification of existing institutional criteria for promotion, or attempt to fit advocacy into a service pathway for promotion. Some advocates will create an AP with the hope that it will be recognized by the promotions committee. As early adopters, various School of Medicine Departments of Pediatrics have also begun to integrate advocacy into promotion tracks to various degrees, examples of which have been highlighted previously[38] and are described here. We are seeing a historical trajectory similar to that seen in medical education, where gradual changes lead to establishment of advocacy as scholarship in its own right: as a fourth pillar supporting institutional missions.

Next Steps for Advocacy Portfolios

APs will undoubtedly go through an evolution similar to Educator Portfolios. Such steps will likely include different versions depending on career stage, such as a developmental AP that allows early advocates to develop career goals versus a promotional

AP that is a summative tool for advocacy work already accomplished.[38,39] It is likely that formats for APs will vary by institution according to values and priorities. Although currently available templates are based on expert consensus, there is a need for more widespread consensus surrounding how advocacy can be measured and displayed as scholarly using an AP.

Consensus on evaluation of advocacy portfolios as scholarship
A method for evaluating advocacy activities as scholarship will be necessary to use APs in the promotion process. Such a tool would allow for peer review of the AP during promotion to determine acceptance as a scholarly product. During the evolution of teaching as scholarship, Schulman and colleagues defined scholarship as works "made public, available for peer review and critique according to accepted standards, and able to be reproduced and built on by other scholars.[23,40] Such a definition allows for the evaluation of unpublished yet "publicly observable" scholarly products in congruence with peer-reviewed scholarly products[41] (eg, white papers in the case of advocacy scholarship).

The challenge here is how to develop sufficient institutional expertise to apply standardized criteria to evaluation of APs. One historical solution to this has been the development of national bodies that would evaluate and certify APs as scholarship. The National Review Board for the Scholarship of Engagement was formed in 2000, whose members are "leaders in the institutionalization of community engagement, service learning, and professional service," and use publicly available criteria for evaluation of the scholarship of engagement.[35] Such approaches are innovative but not sustainable; the true solution would be to increase advocacy training for both faculty and trainees to generate more physicians with the interest and expertise to evaluate these internally.

Assessing the academic value of advocacy scholarly products
Consensus regarding how advocacy is valued by institutions is key to this debate. Whereas research generates "academic currency" in the form of grants and peer-reviewed publications and educators generate academic currency in the form of teaching evaluations, curriculum development, and workshops, there is not yet a standard accepted currency for advocacy. We could consider this currency to be generation of legislative testimony, white papers, and/or community partnerships; yet applying such constraints fails to recognize the full scope of value added by academic advocates.

Both research and medical education have widely accepted standards of value assigned to their respective "academic currency," which allow for progression on a promotion track.[3] For example, in research, we consider "levels" of grant funding, journal metrics or impact factor, order of authorship, and level of reputation (regional vs national). For educators, we consider an institutional curriculum to be valued differently than a nationally used and disseminated curriculum. However, how are we assigning value to the academic currency of advocacy? State versus federal congressional testimony? Invited versus voluntary testimony? Audience of a media spot? Readers of a blog post? Number of retweets? Altmetrics somewhat highlight this difference in value added through advocacy,[42] but still fall short as they focus on the product of peer-reviewed work rather than the scholarly process. Both current and future iterations of APs and evaluation tools should account for and value the skillset specific to physician-advocates.[33]

Advocacy scholars will additionally benefit from increased opportunities for "traditional" peer-reviewed scholarship. For example, medical educators have found success using MedEdPORTAL, an online suppository of teaching and learning resources that have undergone a standardized process of design, implementation, evaluation, and subsequent peer review to acknowledge their status as scholarship. Currently available opportunities for peer review of advocacy projects include *Pediatrics* Advocacy Case Studies and AAP Community Access to Child Health Grants. Opportunities could be expanded through such formats as a regular journal supplement or journal that publishes peer-reviewed advocacy projects, or an online repository for peer-reviewed advocacy projects that allows for national dissemination and replication.

The Role of Academic Institutions

Redefining the academic promotions process through the lens of advocacy
Academic institutions now have an opportunity to advance advocacy by leading the paradigm shift in how these efforts are recognized. Institutions may weave advocacy into the traditional pillars of research, education, and clinical care or include advocacy as an academic pillar that is recognized and valued as a scholarly pursuit for an academic pediatrician.[38] Although this is a spectrum and the former may be the simpler route, the authors assert that the latter may lead to greater downstream effects into communities. For example, the advocacy leadership of Dr Hanna-Attisha on the Flint lead crisis could be viewed as evidence of *National Leadership* a traditional promotion system. Yet without peer-reviewed publication, it would not be recognized as *scholarship* even though these efforts have had a profound impact on the health of Flint children and a downstream effect on lead policy across the country.[9] If faculty are able to clearly delineate the academic path within advocacy, greater impact on the field will likely be generated.

To achieve this, institutions must align their promotions and tenure guidelines with mission-driven goals by valuing alternative forms of scholarship. A case study is provided by the Duke University School of Medicine Appointments, Promotion and Tenure (APT) (**Box 1**). In this approach, faculty select between research, clinical, and education as an area of primary focus, but may use the definitions of alternative scholarship to fulfill scholarly output requirements. Additional examples are highlighted by Bode and colleagues.[38] The recognition of advocacy as alternative or nontraditional scholarship is a wonderful beginning, but more will be necessary to realize the full potential, as highlighted in **Box 2**. Ultimately, early adopters of APs as promotional tools will only be successful if the format is recognized within their respective institutions.

Valuing the Contributions of Academic Advocates
In early 2022, a survey of pediatric department chairs indicated that advocacy has had an increasing importance in the past several years and will continue to increase in importance in the years to come.[43] The vast majority (86%) of pediatric department chairs indicated that advocacy, particularly community engagement, was important to their department's mission.[43] In addition, the majority believed that advocacy was important or very important, in terms of faculty career advancement and promotion. The authors conclude that "given the shift described by the survey respondents toward inclusion of advocacy as a pillar in the overall missions of pediatric departments, the work of advocacy should accordingly be weighted equally in recognition of academic scholarship for promotion alongside traditional areas of clinical, research, and education."[43] Valuing the contributions of physician-advocates also involves recognizing the role this work plays in professional achievement, career satisfaction, and well-being.[44,45] Alternatively, disproportionate value placed on certain types

Box 1
Case Study from the Duke University School of Medicine Appointments, Promotion, and Tenure

Duke University School of Medicine Case Study[49]

In 2020, the Duke School of Medicine (SOM) Appointments, Promotion, and Tenure (APT) committee developed a new framework that *broadened the definition of scholarship* to be inclusive of nontraditional forms, initially including the scholarship of digital work and team science. Advocacy faculty from the Departments of Pediatrics and Community and Family Medicine met with Departmental APT leadership and the School of Medicine APT leadership to discuss *how advocacy could also fit into this broadened definition of scholarship.* Advocates were strongly supported by all leadership to create guidance for the APT process. Drawing from Nerlinger and colleagues,[22] these faculty developed materials to describe *expectations, requirements, and documentation to support the evaluation of advocacy as nontraditional scholarship.* By January 2021, advocacy was included as one of the areas of nontraditional scholarship. Throughout this process, these faculty members used some of the tips and strategies highlighted in **Box 2**, "Advocating for Advocacy."

Within the Duke framework, *advocacy scholarship is defined* as "scholarly activity that promotes the social, economic, educational, and political changes that ameliorate threats to human health and advance the well-being of people."[1] As with traditional scholarship, work cited is required to highlight *quality, quantity, and impact*[32] as well as *evidence of a scholarly approach* through the application of the previously described Glassick framework. The scholar should *identify advocacy-specific scholarly areas for impact* such as non-peer-reviewed content including coauthorship of policy statements/legislative briefs/consensus statements, legislative testimony, development of public health initiatives that become standard of care, participation in local and regional task forces, and establishment of community partnerships. *Ability to obtain funding for advocacy efforts* (eg, grant funding for community partnered programs, funding for educational efforts, funding for health equity programs) or to have a key role in securing funding for multidisciplinary and/or interprofessional teams is also considered scholarship.

Examples Based on the Level of Appointment

Associate Professor

- The Associate Professor is expected to have an established record in advocacy engagement, knowledge dissemination, community outreach, advocacy teaching/mentoring, and/or advocacy leadership/administration.
- Expected to have leadership responsibilities in institutional, local, and regional organizations that promote advocacy and community engagement.
- Effective mentoring of trainees and junior faculty is expected, within the sphere of practice of the faculty member.

Professor

- Faculty at the rank of Professor will have an established record for advocacy engagement, knowledge dissemination, community outreach, advocacy teaching/mentoring, and/or advocacy leadership/administration.
- Scholarly contributions in advocacy should result in impact, locally, and/or nationally.
- Faculty at this rank are expected to have leadership positions in local and regional medical or community partnered organizations, national accreditation organizations, scholarly societies, departmental advocacy committees, relevant school of medicine or department committees, and/or national advocacy or health equity organizations

Future Directions

- *Institutional Professional Development on Use of Advocacy Portfolios:* Paradigm shift requires both shared terminology and mentorship to create momentum. At Duke, advocacy faculty within pediatrics are currently engaged to provide education across the department and at the level of the SOM APT to ensure that all faculty understand how the scholarly impact of advocacy work is articulated and valued in the APT process.
- *Professional Development Resource Library:* Additional professional support for advocacy faculty could be created through a shared institutional library of intellectual development statements, CVs, and advocacy portfolios to support faculty in their own APT process.
- *Broadened Definition of Support for Promotion:* Institutions can consider broadening the scope of support for promotion of academic advocates by accepting letters from leaders of community coalitions, policymakers, and other community partners.

Box 2
Tips for advocating for advocacy within one's institution

Advocating for Advocacy: Tips and Strategies
1. Learn more about local, regional, and national professional development opportunities
   - Join regional and national groups such as the American Academy of Pediatrics (AAP) Community Pediatrics Training Initiative, or Academic Pediatric Association (APA) Advocacy Training Special Interest Group, or apply for the APA Health Policy Scholars Program.
   - Participate in workgroups (Professional Development and Leadership).
   - Partner with your AAP state chapter to create an advocacy special interest group or to network and identify other advocates.
2. Identify your local network and infrastructure
   - Does your department have an advocacy chair or other recognized advocacy leadership roles?
   - Who in your department or division is involved in advocacy work?
   - What resources exist to support faculty advocacy work within your department?
3. Tell your advocacy story
   - Discuss with leadership whether Advocacy Portfolios are recognized in promotion versus adding advocacy sections to CV.
   - Start developing a personal Advocacy Portfolio and advocacy professional development statement.
4. Learn about where advocacy fits within your institution
   - What is your local Appointments, Promotion, and Tenure structure? Is the work of advocacy recognized?
   - Who would you talk to on your promotions committee to reexamine promotion criteria in light of new processes, leaning on examples from other institutions who have recognized advocacy as scholarship?
   - Is advocacy identified in your institutional mission? How can you use this to help show the value of advocacy work?
5. Understand facilitators and motivators for gaining alignment between institutional leadership and those practicing advocacy
   - How can you identify and help address leadership knowledge gaps surrounding advocacy as scholarship?
   - How can the experience and expertise of early adopters be used to help inform leadership?
   - How can you help facilitate discussion between early adopters and key Appointments, Promotion, and Tenure leadership at your institution?

---

of scholarship serves to perpetuate inequities in faculty recognition and advancement.[6]

The dedication of resources through time, funding, and training is one way that academic institutions and departments of pediatrics can begin to recognize the value of advocacy scholarship. Traditionally, a researcher is given resources (ie, time) to pursue grant funding and research activities that benefit the health of patients and populations. We proposed that academic advocates should be given similar resources to pursue the improvement of policies that benefit the health of communities as well. Conducting advocacy work, developing skills specific to physician advocates, and training and mentoring the next generation of physicians in advocacy practices[7] all require time, similar to research and education. Leadership positions for advocacy can serve as a conduit for the development of such programs.

We acknowledge that professional organization alignment with this definition of scholarship is imperative as well. This includes recognizing advocacy scholarly products in graduate medical education and awarding pediatrician credit for Maintenance of Certification in advocacy, both of which are areas actively under development.[7]

There is also an opportunity to build a national academic advocacy community to support and enhance faculty development. The AAP CPTI is poised to do just that through their development of a national steering committee to support the scholarship of advocacy. Specifically, the leadership and career development pillar aims to organize, enhance, and promote resources that work to foster the growth and success of pediatricians focused on advocacy. Early work of this group includes the development of a professional resource repository with examples of advocacy-related job descriptions, CVs, personal statements, and ultimately APs.[37]

Valuing the health of populations

The shift to value-based care, with health care institutions bearing financial risk for a population of patients, offers a timely policy window through which to frame a paradigm shift in academics. Health care systems in value-based contracts are responsible for reducing inappropriate health care utilization through the prevention of illness and improving equity in health outcomes. All of these motivators have produced a renewed focus on community-integrated solutions to move health care upstream by addressing social determinants of health (SDoH). Advocacy efforts align with such priorities, yet unless they result in a peer-reviewed publication or grant, may not be recognized in proportion to their importance, or impact on a practical level in traditional academic promotion systems.

Such is the reality of disconnect currently between the actions of health care systems and the mission, vision, and values of the academic institutions with which they are associated. This apparent discrepancy can be reconciled through a similar focus on community health and equity as drivers, particularly within the promotion process. The writings of Boyer and Glassick serve to reiterate how faculty pursuit of scholarship should align with institutional missions; if hospitals and medical academic institutions are dedicated to improving the health of communities, promotion pathways should reflect the value added of advocacy work that is critical to achieving this aim.[6]

Advocacy work also aligns with health care system engagement with communities through a variety of mechanisms including relevance to:

- The process of screening for SDoH and partnering with communities to address positive screens
- The role of health care systems as anchor institutions to improve community health and well-being[46]
- The integration of community into clinical care, education, and research to build community trust and improve equity[47]
- Community benefit and community health needs assessment requirements for nonprofit hospitals to maintain tax-exempt status[5]

Physicians can also have a direct impact through cooperation with institutional government affairs offices. Many health care institutions have an advocacy presence at the local, state, and federal level. Examples include Ohio Children's Hospital Association, Children's National Hospital's Child Health Advocacy Institute,[5] and Nemours Children's Health National Office of Policy and Prevention. Such mechanisms have the potential to provide infrastructure and resources for physician advocacy to be valued at the institutional level.

SUMMARY

Although the authors discuss the role of APs as a developmental and promotional tool in academic medical settings, this format can be applied outside of this setting for purposes such as gaining leadership support for advocacy work in the form of funding or time, support for financial bonus, or application for health policy or advocacy positions. Although our discussion surrounds the role of physicians, these arguments are relevant to many different types of clinicians who might be undergoing the appointment, promotion, and tenure process, or who desire to be recognized for the value their advocacy work adds to the institutional mission.

Future goals include the expansion of this framework not only beyond pediatrics but also beyond medical institutions. Schools of medicine can also benefit from the learning and resources of nonmedical institutions of higher learning, such as the Research University Civic Engagement Network, established in 2008 to "advance civic engagement and engaged scholarship among [R-1] research universities."[48] If academic medical centers are dedicated to improving health, it makes sense to recognize advocacy scholarship, as many other institutions of higher learning are already doing in the form of scholarship of engagement.

Shifting the focus of faculty promotion from *scholarly product* to *scholarly process* will allow for adoption of advocacy as a pillar of academic institutional missions. Faculty who align advocacy work with the institutional mission, conduct advocacy projects in a scholarly manner, and disseminate this work for colleagues' inspection should realize congruence in the academic promotion and evaluation process. To help achieve such congruence, **Box 2** outlines steps to "advocate for advocacy" throughout one's journey as an academic advocate, from identifying professional development opportunities to impacting institutional promotion processes. Such actions by early adopters will allow advocates to continue charting a path forward, leading to widespread adoption of advocacy as scholarship.

The overarching goal is for academic institutions to reexamine and redefine how they value the scholarly contributions of faculty in the context of community health and equity. Pediatricians have the potential to act as agents of change to improve the health and well-being of children and communities; this potential can only be fully realized with support from leadership, institutions, and organizations. We as pediatric advocates need to be the ones telling our stories that are so critical to our purpose, profession, and patients.

DISCLOSURE

All authors have no conflicts of interest to disclose.

REFERENCES

1. Earnest MA, Wong SL, Federico SG. Physician advocacy: What is it and how do we do it? Acad Med 2010;85:6367.

2. Oberg CN. Pediatric advocacy: yesterday, today, and tomorrow. Pediatrics 2003 Aug;112(2):406–9.

3. Gros L, Kenneth RR. Evolving the Faculty Reward System. Acad Med Sept 2000; 75(9):868–9.

4. Institute of Medicine (US). In: Kohn LT, editor. Committee on the roles of academic health centers in the 21st Century. Academic health centers: leading change in the 21st century. . Washington (DC): National Academies Press; 2004. Accessed May 5, 2022.

5. Wright JL, Morris AM. Child health advocacy in the academic medical center. Pediatr Ann 2007;36(10):637–43.

6. Boyer EL. In: Moser D, Ream TC, Braxton JM, editors. Scholarship Reconsidered: priorities of the Professoriate. expanded edition. San Francisco: Jossey-Bass; 2016.

7. Nerlinger A, Shah A. Faculty Support for Advocacy is Key to Training the Next Generation of Pediatrician-Advocates. Hosp Pediatr 2022;12(6):e223–4.

8. Gruen RL, Campbell EG, Blumenthal D. Public roles of US physicians: community participation, political involvement, and collective advocacy. JAMA 2006;296(20): 2467–75.

9. Hanna-Attisha M. What the Eyes Don't See: a story of crisis, Resistance, and hope in an American city. New York: One World; 2019.

10. MLive. Hurley doctor recommends switching away from Flint River water [video]. YouTube. 2015. Available at: https://www.youtube.com/watch?v=6tELb594WTw. Accessed May 24, 2022.

11. Jenco M. AAP denounces federal initiative separating families at the border. AAP News. 2018. Available at: https://publications.aap.org/aapnews/news/6615. Accessed May 24, 2022.

12. Kraft C. Letter to the US Secretary of Homeland Security. Authored March 1. 2018. Available at: https://downloads.aap.org/DOFA/AAP%20Letter%20to%20DHS%20Secretary%2003-01-18.pdf. Accessed May 24, 2022.

13. Schering S. Pediatricians seek state, federal offices to give children a voice. AAP News. 2022. Available at: https://publications.aap.org/aapnews/news/19998/Pediatricians-seek-state-federal-offices-to-give. Accessed May 24, 2022.

14. Howell BA, Kristal RB, Whitmire LR, et al. A Systematic Review of Advocacy Curricula in Graduate Medical Education. J Gen Intern Med 2019;34(11): 2592–601.

15. Chimonas S, Mamoor M, Kaltenboeck A, et al. The future of physician advocacy: a survey of US medical students. BMC Med Educ 2021;21(1):399.

16. Blankenburg R, Poitevien P, Gonzalez Del Rey J, et al. Dismantling Racism: Association of Pediatric Program Directors; Commitment to Action. Acad Pediatr 2020;20(8):1051–3.

17. Jindal M, Heard-Garris N, Empey A, et al. Getting "Our House" in Order: Re-Building Academic Pediatrics by Dismantling the Anti-Black Racist Foundation. Acad Pediatr 2020;20(8):1044–50.

18. Orr CJ, Montez KG, Omoruyi EA, et al. Implementing What We Preach: Anti-Racist Recommendations from the Academic Pediatric Association Leadership Development Nomination Committee Task Force. Acad Pediatr 2022;22(3):356–9.

19. Winthrop ZA, Michelson CD, Nash KA. Training the Next Generation of Pediatrician-Advocates: A New Focus on the Inpatient Setting. Hosp Pediatr 2021;11(10):e266–9.

20. Huddle T. Medical professionalism and medical education should not involve commitments to political advocacy. Acad Med 2011;86:378–83.

21. Dobson S, Voyer S, Regehr G. Agency and activism: Rethinking health advocacy in the medical profession. Acad Med 2012;87:1161–4.

22. Nerlinger AL, Shah AN, Beck AF, et al. The Advocacy Portfolio: A Standardized Tool for Documenting Physician Advocacy. Acad Med 2018;93(6):860–8.

23. Glassick CE. Boyer's expanded definitions of scholarship, the standards for assessing scholarship, and the elusiveness of the scholarship of teaching. Acad Med 2000;75:877–80.

24. The Carnegie Foundation for the Advancement of Teaching. The Condition of the Professoriate: attitudes and Trends. Princeton, NJ: Carnegie Foundation for the

Advancement of Teaching; 1989. Available at: https://eric.ed.gov/?id=ED312963. Accessed May 3, 2022.

25. Glassick CE, Huber MT, Maeroff GI. Scholarship Assessed: evaluation of the Professoriate. 1st edition. San Francisco: Jossey-Bass; 1997.

26. Gusic M, Chandran L, Balmer D, et al. Educator portfolio template of the academic pediatric associations' education scholars program. MedEdPORTAL 2007;3:626. https://doi.org/10.15766/mep_2374-8265.626. Accessed November 27, 2017.

27. Simpson D, Fincher RM, Hafler JP, et al. Advancing educators and education by defining the components and evidence associated with educational scholarship. Med Educ 2007;41:1002–9.

28. Baldwin C, Chandran L, Gusic M. Guidelines for evaluating the educational performance of medical school faculty: Priming a national conversation. Teach Learn Med 2011;23:285–97.

29. Gusic ME, Baldwin CD, Chandran L, et al. Evaluating educators using a novel toolbox: Applying rigorous criteria flexibly across institutions. Acad Med 2014; 89:1006–11.

30. Chandran L, Gusic M, Baldwin C, et al. APA educator portfolio analysis tool. MedEdPORTAL 2009;5:1659. Available at: https://www.mededportal.org/publication/1659. Accessed November 27, 2017.

31. Chandran L, Gusic M, Baldwin C, et al. Evaluating the performance of medical educators: A novel analysis tool to demonstrate the quality and impact of educational activities. Acad Med 2009;84:58–66.

32. Gusic M, Amiel J, Baldwin C, et al. Using the AAMC Toolbox for evaluating educators: You be the judge. MedEdPORTAL 2013;9:9313. https://doi.org/10.15766/mep_2374- 8265.9313. Accessed November 27, 2017.

33. Dobson S, Voyer S, Hubinette M, et al. From the clinic to the community: The activities and abilities of effective health advocates. Acad Med 2015;90:214–20.

34. Driscoll A, Lynton EA. Making outreach visible: a guide to documenting professional service and outreach. Washington, DC: American Association for Higher Education; 1999. Available at: https://eric.ed.gov/?id=ED441392. Accessed May 3, 2022.

35. Driscoll A, Sandman L. From Maverick to Mainstream: The Scholarship of Engagement. J Higher Education Outreach Engagement 2016;20(1):83.

36. Bringle R, Malloy E, Games R, editors. Colleges and universities as Citizens. 1st edition. Boston: Allyn & Bacon; 1999.

37. American Academy of Pediatrics. American Academy of Pediatrics Community Pediatrics Training Initiative. 2021. Available at: https://www.aap.org/cpti. Accessed May 3, 2022.

38. Bode S, Hoffman BD, Chapman S, et al. Academic Careers in Advocacy: Aligning Institutional Values through Use of an Advocacy Portfolio. Pediatrics 2022; 150(1):e2021055014.

39. Baldwin CD, Gusic M, Chandran L. The Educator Portfolio: A Tool for Career Development. Association of American Medical Colleges. September 23, 2010. Available at: https://www.aamc.org/professional-development/affinity-groups/gfa/faculty-vitae/educator-portfolio-tool. Accessed May 24, 2022.

40. Shulman L. The Scholarship of Teaching. Change 1999;31(5):11.

41. Braxton JM, Luckey W, Helland P. Institutionalizing a broader View of scholarship through Boyer's four domains. San Francisco: Jossey-Bass; 2002.

42. Galligan F, Dyas-Correia S. Altmetrics: Rethinking the Way We Measure. Serials Rev 2013;39(1):56–61.

43. Chung RJ, Ramirez MR, Best DL, et al. Advocacy and Community Engagement: Perspectives from Pediatric Department Chairs. J Pediatr 2022;248:6.e3–10.e3.

44. Webber S, Babal JC, Shadman KA, et al. Exploring Academic Pediatrician Perspectives of Factors Impacting Physician Well-Being. Acad Pediatr 2020;20(6): 833–9.

45. Dodson NA, Talib HJ, Gao Q, et al. Pediatricians as Child Health Advocates: The Role of Advocacy Education. Health Prom Pract 2021;22(1):13–7.

46. Weston MJ, Pham BH, Zuckerman D. Building Community Well-being by Leveraging the Economic Impact of Health Systems. Nurs Adm Q 2020;44(3): 215–20.

47. Alberti PM, Sutton KM, Cooper LA, et al. Communities, Social Justice, and Academic Health Centers. Acad Med 2018;93(1):20–4.

48. The Research University Civic Engagement Network (TRUCEN). 2021. Available at: https://compact.org/trucen/. Accessed June 13, 2022.

49. Best D, Maradiaga Panayotti GM, Martinez-Bianchi V. Duke University School of Medicine Appointment, Promotion, and Tenure Advocacy Scholarship Framework. Available at: https://medschool.duke.edu/sites/default/files/2021-05/advocacy_scholarship_framework_0.pdf. Accessed June 14, 2022.

Making Advocacy Part of Your Job

Working for Children in Any Practice Setting

Lee Savio Beers, MD[a],*, Melinda A. Williams-Willingham, MD[b],
Lisa J. Chamberlain, MD, MPH[c]

KEYWORDS

- Advocacy • Child health • Legislative advocacy • Community advocacy
- Medical education

KEY POINTS

- Effective health advocacy can improve child health at the individual and population levels.
- Advocacy is part of a standard of professional practice; child health advocacy provides a fundamental foundation for health care and is supported by the development of educational curriculum for teaching advocacy.
- Leveraging the strengths and understanding the limitations of one's pediatric practice setting can make child health advocacy more effective and rewarding.
- A scarcity of time and resources is a common barrier for child health advocates, which can be addressed by a number of practical strategies.

INTRODUCTION

Effective child health advocacy is essential to advance goals for improving child health. Advocacy can improve access to equitable care and "… promotes those social, economic, educational, and political changes that ameliorate the suffering and threats to human health and well-being," thus advancing overall health.[1] However, although advocacy has been a part of pediatrics since its origins as a specialty, many barriers to engaging in health advocacy exist, which can be challenging to navigate across a variety of practice settings. Pediatrics as a specialty was recognized in

Note: Dr Beers' contributions as an author were not as an official representative of the American Academy of Pediatrics (AAP) and do not represent the official position of the Board of Directors of the AAP.
[a] Child Health Advocacy Institute, Children's National Hospital, 111 Michigan Avenue Northwest, Washington, DC 20010, USA; [b] InTouch Pediatrics, 2321 Henry Clower Boulevard, Suite A, Snellville, GA 30078, USA; [c] Department of Pediatrics, Stanford, School of Medicine, 453 Quarry Road, Mail Code 5459, Stanford, CA 94305, USA
* Corresponding author.
E-mail address: lbeers@childrensnational.org

the early twentieth century because of the vision of a group of physicians with the conviction that children and their diseases require special attention by those skilled in their care.[2] This conviction led to many advancements and an understanding of the importance of exacting standards of child health. Physicians who cared for children were now unified with a shared goal.[3] Indeed, the founding of the American Academy of Pediatrics (AAP) grew out of a recognition in the 1920s that these goals did not align with the position of the American Medical Association (AMA) on the Sheppard-Towner Act, which would have provided federal funds to establish programs focused on improving maternal and infant health. The AMA Section on Pediatrics strongly supported this Act despite opposition from others within the organization, which largely stemmed from concerns around the role of the federal government in health care. This advocacy led to the reprimand of the Section by the AMA, and was ultimately the impetus to form a national pediatric society. In June 1930, the name AAP and a constitution for the fledgling organization were adopted.[4]

Advocacy as a Professional Standard

Many challenges and opportunities requiring advocacy lie ahead for pediatricians in this rapidly changing world; however, there are clear barriers to becoming an effective pediatrician-advocate. Lack of time, inadequate training and mentorship, lack of resources, and the length of time it may take to successfully resolve an advocacy issue can dissuade some pediatricians from engagement. In addition, pediatricians can and should play a key role in communicating the needs of children based on evidenced-based research; however, this requires public trust, something which has been affected by the complexity and public disagreement around the response to the COVID-19 pandemic.[5] Furthermore, controversial issues, if not carefully navigated, can affect not only the financial health of one's institution or private practice but also the emotional well-being of the pediatrician.[6] These contextual factors emphasize the critical importance of fostering a culture of nonpartisan advocacy and the engagement of pediatricians from a wide range of communities, specialties, and practice settings.

Advocacy provides a fundamental foundation for health care and is supported by the development of educational curriculum for teaching advocacy. The Accreditation Council for Graduate Medical Education (ACGME) has formally included advocacy in the Common Program Requirements for pediatric residency programs[7] but the content and depth of advocacy curricula vary widely.[8] Comprehensive training curricula are essential to fulfill ACGME requirements and support the acquisition of the requisite knowledge and skills to be an effective physician advocate. After graduation, time for professional advocacy work should be permitted and encouraged to catalyze change to meet the needs of today's children.

Facilitators and Barriers to Integrating Advocacy into Your Practice

There are a wide range of organizational practice settings, which are each accompanied by unique strengths and limitations relevant to physician advocacy. The strategies used and infrastructure available to support such activities also varies widely. First, we define "organizational settings" and then will explore the range of advocacy opportunities that exist.

Pediatric practice settings span outpatient to inpatient, and from solo practitioners to large groups. Here, we define 3 general categories, although recognize that not every practice setting fits neatly into one of these categorizations: (1) independent private practice; (2) outpatient publicly funded practices, such as those found in Federally Qualified Health Centers, county-based clinics or health systems, and some community academic practices; and (3) large group (or group-like) practices, such as large multidisciplinary or pediatric "supergroups," Health Maintenance Organizations (HMOs), and nonprofit academic health systems that provide both inpatient and outpatient care. There are also various types of advocacy, including (1) individual level advocacy, where the focus of effort is to assist one patient at a time; (2) community advocacy, where attention to elicit change is at the level of a unified group, which can be defined by geography, faith, cultural background, or other unique factors; (3) organization level advocacy, where change is sought within the system of care or practice; and (4) governmental advocacy, where the focus of change is at the level of decision-makers who create and pass legislation. In this article, we will focus on how pediatricians can advance the well-being of children within their care organization, whatever the setting and regardless of payer mix, and inclusive of both inpatient and outpatient settings. Although each practice setting has unique considerations, organizational assets and strengths can typically support the pediatrician to effectively advocate for the health of children and families.

Although each individual practice or organization has its own strengths and limitations, there are some generally common experiences within each category worth noting. Many pediatricians see patients within an independent practice or group practice setting, which has many advocacy strengths. Although it can vary depending on practice and/or group size and complexity, the ability to be nimble and respond to time-sensitive issues is an asset often found in independent practices, which typically lack the layers of bureaucracy found in county or university-based clinics. Larger pediatric "supergroups" can sometimes represent several hundred pediatricians and other pediatric health providers, increasing their capacity to be an influential voice. The limitations of advocating in such a setting include a lack of incentive structure that rewards advocacy engagement, and less buffering from pushback when advocating on issues that may be controversial or sensitive within the practice's community. Additionally, settings of any kind with a large percentage of families experiencing food insecurity, housing instability, inadequately funded schools, systemic racism, and other barriers to health often recognize an acute need for physician advocacy. However, this elevated urgency and motivation to act can be stymied in publicly funded practice settings that may have strict restrictions regarding engaging in advocacy. Finally, large academic or health-system–owned groups similarly have inherent tradeoffs. The advocacy strengths of these settings may include extant infrastructure of government relations professionals and departments that have expertise in health-care policy. They enjoy name recognition due to being a regional and/or state anchor institution with inherent political influence, and leadership, including board membership, and are often "grass tops" influencers. The advocacy limitations in this setting often include nonprofit, 501(c)3 status, which limits the amount of lobbying that can be done, occasional conflicting priorities, and increased bureaucracy. Although there is no "perfect" setting for pediatric advocacy, knowing the strengths and limitations of one's individual practice allows pediatricians to leverage support and to pivot and make use of adjacent structures in order to address barriers.

The scarcity of time, which ultimately is the result of competing priorities, exists across all settings. Alignment of incentives varies across settings, with advocacy being increasingly supported for promotion consideration in many academic settings.[9] Advocacy and local engagement can also increase the strength of the relationship that the pediatrician or health system has with their surrounding community, which can then indirectly lead to improved physician–patient relationships, increased patient volume and more opportunities to partner with families or other local organizations to improve care. There is often also alignment around increased community and policy engagement for regions that have moved to an accountable care organization (ACO) payment structure.[10] Advancing conversations of alternative payment structures that meet the needs of children, families, and pediatricians[11] will be key to ultimately moving all pediatric organizations, regardless of structure, to an upstream, preventive model that deeply embraces advocacy and equity.

Advocacy Strategies Across Practice Settings

Pediatricians can adopt strategies to advance advocacy goals that are practical across a wide range of practice settings. Some of the most common strategies include education, policy or regulatory change, and community engagement. Education is at the heart of successful advocacy, helping others to more deeply understand the "how" and the "why" of proposed changes, and increase motivation to act. Educational efforts can be targeted toward those with the authority and ability to make change (eg, legislators or administrators), toward colleagues with the intent of engaging them as allies, or toward the public with the goal of increasing public attention on an issue in order to facilitate change. These types of efforts often occur both in formal medical educational settings and informal community settings (eg, schools), as well as in the legislature and the media. Pediatricians in all practice settings can effectively engage in education in each of these ways; however—while it is difficult to fully generalize—the ease of opportunity and perceived value may differ. For example, pediatricians in academic settings may have more built-in opportunities to teach in formal settings (eg, Grand Rounds, resident conferences) and greater perceived value of these opportunities due to their contribution to academic promotion. Alternately, pediatricians in independent practice may have closer relationships to the resources and services in their communities, and thus more opportunity to provide education in community-based settings. Larger institutions may have established public relations departments who can facilitate media opportunities; however, a pediatrician who is trusted with close ties to their community may more easily develop the relationships to become the "go to" resource for local journalists.

Policy and regulatory change can occur external to an organization (eg, local or federal government), or internal to an organization (eg, health system policies and procedures). Medical societies, such as the AAP, and institutional government affairs specialists can help facilitate opportunities to engage with legislators on a particular issue. Although sometimes the "weight' of an institution can bring prestige or visibility to an issue, the trust and credibility of a community-based pediatrician is highly valued, and their experiences caring for patients provide essential insight. Internal health system changes can also be extremely impactful and, often, can be more easily and nimbly implemented at a smaller practice or organization.

Regardless of organizational setting, partnering and engaging with families and communities enhances the effectiveness by amplifying important messages and contributing to shared learning. Most importantly, it promotes equity through centering the voices of those most affected by an issue.[12] Pediatricians should seek ways to authentically engage with, contribute to, and learn from the communities where they practice. In addition to the essential commitment to community engagement, other organizational partnerships can amplify momentum toward impactful and lasting change. Professionals and/or organizations such as local medical societies, family run organizations, legal advocacy groups, and local leaders can all contribute skills and knowledge, and may provide an additional avenue for the pediatrician to engage in advocacy outside of their practice setting. A number of these partnership types deserve special mention given their accessibility and potential to provide important supports regardless of practice setting. As noted, medical societies can provide support with legislative advocacy but also can offer other advocacy and skill-building opportunities and are readily accessible to any pediatrician in practice. Both national and local medical societies offer great value, and many national groups have affiliated local chapters, which further enhance this value. For pediatricians who have a specific area of interest, local or national nonprofits may provide additional opportunities for support and engagement. Many of these organizations have a particular focus on a content area (eg, environmental health) or specific population (eg, immigrant families). For pediatricians who practice in larger settings, government affairs specialists may be available for support and should, at a minimum, be made aware of any advocacy efforts being undertaken by those who work in their health system.

Addressing Barriers and Special Considerations

Time and resources are among the most commonly cited barriers to engaging in advocacy.[1,13] As noted, by leveraging partnerships and membership in medical societies pediatricians can share responsibilities and collectively contribute to advocacy efforts. As the old saying goes, "many hands make light work." For medical professionals, this is particularly important because the intensity of patient care, which must be prioritized, can ebb and flow and affect one's ability to actively engage in advocacy during any given period of time. However, joining with other professionals can effectively provide the structure and support to address many of the drivers of health disparities, which might otherwise seem intractable. Investing in building relationships over time will make this type of collaborative advocacy easier and more seamless.

Partnerships can also provide opportunities to seek philanthropic or government funding to attain additional support, including offsetting some of the pediatricians' time to do nonclinical work. Although this more commonly happens in academic settings, there are many local philanthropic or medical society funding opportunities that are readily available to pediatricians in smaller or independent practices. Although they tend to be smaller in amount, they also may have less burdensome application and reporting requirements.

A more vexing and complex barrier is navigating progressively more polarized political environments. Many important child health issues, such as immunizations, the response to the COVID-19 pandemic, and care for transgender youth have become increasingly charged social issues at the center of intense political debate. Pediatricians who engage in advocacy on these types of issues may face personal and sometimes vicious verbal or online attacks, or attacks targeted at their workplace, and rarely may even have their personal safety put at risk. The state and local political environment can heavily influence a pediatrician's experience as a health advocate. Pediatricians may experience ethical conflict if they want to speak up on an issue their health system has chosen not to engage with, or holds a differing viewpoint on. In rare cases, one's employment may be in jeopardy if they speak out on a politically charged issue. There are no easy solutions, circumstances can be very individualized, and the environment is rapidly changing. Pediatricians are encouraged to seek advice and support from medical societies, their institutions, and/or their mentors to aid them in navigating these difficult issues when needed. Often these resources can provide important peer support, or offer an opportunity to leverage the expertise, experience, and influence of a larger organization or institution to decrease vulnerability of the individual or a smaller practice.

Several practice settings have unique barriers, which confront the pediatrician advocate. In university or other academic settings, career growth and advancement is typically tied to academic productivity, which has traditionally been defined by research and education scholarship. Although health advocacy is increasingly being recognized as scholarship in and of itself,[9] more frequently pediatricians who engage in health advocacy must either look for ways to translate their activities into traditional academic currency or accept a slower career trajectory. Similarly, subspecialists who are interested in health advocacy may have difficulty finding academic collaborators or networks who share their interests. Finally, pediatricians who work in local, state, or federal government roles as well as uniformed pediatricians have significant limitations on the types of advocacy strategies they can use in the context of their professional position. These groups very often need to participate in their advocacy activities outside the workplace and with clear divisions between acting in their personal, as opposed to professional, capacity. For each of these groups, medical societies can be important assets, helping to provide leadership and networking opportunities, and allowing pediatricians to contribute to health advocacy in ways that are not in conflict with their professional limitations or obligations.

The Value of Engaging in Child Health Advocacy

Ultimately, improved child health is the key value and goal of all child health advocacy; although advocacy is at the core of the profession of pediatrics, the pandemic brought this value into even more acute focus. Long-standing and pervasive health disparities, which have been highlighted over the course of both the pandemic and concomitant increased attention to systemic racism, have challenged our nation and pediatrics to transform our existing practices—which often fail to promote health equity for all children. Despite the challenges, we have also seen many encouraging successes. Pre-existing commitment to addressing equity and systemic racism in health care, as well as infrastructure supporting long-standing, community partnerships, allowed some institutions to respond with support that mitigated the dual challenge of the pandemic and the overdue reckoning of racial justice.[14] Partnerships between pediatric health systems and local food banks, school districts, and core service agencies that provide housing and employment support were all critical to mobilize new resources and capacity in a time of crisis. These types of responses are incentivized by shifts to ACO models that prioritize outcomes at the population level.

There are additional benefits common to all types of practice settings to engaging in child health advocacy, be they independent small groups or large health systems: physician satisfaction, improved physician recruitment, and enhanced reputation. There is emerging evidence that engaging in advocacy improves professional satisfaction and decreases burnout in pediatricians.[15,16] Increasingly medical students applying to residency and graduating pediatricians entering the workforce place high importance on community engagement and advocacy, and the settings that provide such opportunities have a competitive recruiting advantage. This was articulated in a recent national survey of pediatric department chairs who noted that these activities were increasingly seen as a top priority for their incoming trainees and junior faculty members.[17] There was evidence from the same survey that this trend will only continue: Four out of 5 chairs reported an increasing importance of advocacy in their academic departments compared with 5 years ago and further state the 5 years from now advocacy would be "more" or "much more" important. This suggests that the time to embrace community engagement and advocacy is now.

Case Study: Checking the Vital Signs of the Georgia Medicaid Delivery System for Children.

A 10-year-old boy with Medicaid presented to his pediatrician, who owns an independent small practice, with a 5-day history of pain, swelling, and redness in his left hand. The patient was diagnosed with complicated cellulitis, which required debridement and surgical intervention but was unable to access care in a timely way because there were no hand surgeons in the network who accepted the patient's insurance. Through working together with the state chapter of the AAP to address systemic barriers to care, the patient was ultimately able to get the care he needed, and long-term changes were made that affected many other patients as well.

Problem: Soon after the conversion of substantial portions of state Medicaid enrollees to HMOs began in 2006, pediatricians and the Georgia Chapter of the AAP became concerned about the reduced access to care for children in the Medicaid and PeachCare programs. Moving 750,000 Medicaid children into managed care in the span of just 4 months was unprecedented in the history of the Medicaid programs nationwide. Other factors, namely the implementation of methodologies of income and citizenship verification, changing eligibility requirements and shortcomings in implementation of these new policies resulted in many more children unable to enroll in the Medicaid program, even though eligible by income and citizenship standards. Taken as a whole, these circumstances pointed to a serious lack of access for needed care and poor-quality care for many children in the Medicaid program. The problem, if not addressed directly and aggressively, would worsen. The result would likely be an increased risk to these children of not getting the needed care in a prompt manner, and ballooning ER and hospitalization costs that could have been prevented by a source of stable, ongoing primary care for the child in their medical home.

Recognizing the urgency of the situation, the Georgia Chapter of the AAP conducted a telephone survey to determine the scope of the problem. Pediatric health care providers (such as pediatricians, pediatric specialists, and advanced practice providers) in 11 cities were surveyed and 80 practices responded. Pediatric orthopedists, to whom access had been historically limited, were also surveyed. The survey results confirmed that there was a lack of adequate access in certain parts of the state both for primary care pediatrics and for pediatric specialty care, such as orthopedics.

Solution: Through these networks, a surgical provider for the patient was identified. AAP chapter leadership contacted pediatricians throughout the state to gather additional data, and met with state Care Management Organizations (CMO). The culmination of these efforts led to a framework to assess the implementation of the transition to CMOs.

1. Improve access to primary and specialty care;
2. Improve quality of outcomes—preventive and acute care;
3. Improve the logistics for providers—web portal technology, claims processing, medical management, credentialing, and patient assignment; and
4. Provide adequate payment for providers—amount of payment and contract negotiation process.

Outcome: The patient's CMO agreed to reimburse the hand surgeon adequately to perform the procedure and the patient recovered uneventfully. The pediatrician's practice changed internal processes by adjusting workflows and repurposing staff to assist with coordination of patient care. Importantly, the statewide advocacy efforts were a major catalyst of change. It generated dialog in the community between pediatricians, pediatric subspecialists, hospital systems, managed Medicaid CMOs, and the Georgia Chapter of the AAP, which ultimately led to improved access to quality care. Payment was not the focus of the survey. However, the compilation of patient stories and strong advocacy efforts by pediatricians throughout the state ultimately led to improved payment rates for providers. Although the payment rates did not improve swiftly, action was later taken by the Georgia Legislature to improve payment to Medicare parity for more than 150 billing codes after a decade of ongoing advocacy by pediatricians and the Georgia Chapter of the AAP.

This case study illustrates advocacy in action, highlighting the need for pediatricians to recognize the importance of integrating advocacy into their practice and their ability to implement meaningful change. Sustained advocacy efforts can prevent significant morbidity and mortality to infants, children, and teens, which can result from lack of access to care. In addition, continued advocacy for adequate provider payment rates can be a significant contributor to preventing the erosion of access to care. The use of internal and external resources in this case study led to a culture shift of systems and eventually organizational change.

Lessons Learned

The authors have each successfully integrated child health advocacy into their career across a variety of settings, including small, independent practice, uniformed services, and academic pediatrics, and have developed robust professional networks of other pediatricians who have similarly integrated advocacy into their careers. A review of the literature and reflection on the experiences of colleagues across a wide range of practice settings reveal some important lessons learned.

1. As noted throughout, membership in medical professional organizations such as the AAP offers wide-ranging supports and benefits, including access to collaborators, mentors, and government affairs expertise. The inherent power of many voices speaking in a unified way on an issue is facilitated and amplified through organizational activities and relieves some of the individual time and resource burden. Additionally, for those who desire deeper involvement there are built in leadership opportunities which can be personally very rewarding and contribute to career advancement. For the busy pediatrician, these organizations offer a very effective and efficient way to utilize their passion and expertise to effect change. Health systems should look for ways to support their staff's participation in these types of organizations through financial support for membership dues and supporting the use of nonclinical time for participation in activities.

2. There is no question that having increased time and resources to devote to advocacy activities is beneficial but these supports are typically difficult to access. Funding and grant opportunities, however small, can often provide the breathing room to make the pediatrician advocate more successful. Additionally, emphasizing the value of advocacy for increasing visibility and reputation, positively influencing financing and payment, and increasing professional satisfaction and decreasing burnout may be compelling arguments to encourage leadership in a wide range of practice settings to provide additional time and resources. In not-for-profit health systems, the pediatrician advocate can also contribute to required community-benefit activities, leveraging their interests to support a legal organizational requirement. Increased uptake of the use of an advocacy portfolio for academic promotion will also help drive resources toward scholarly advocacy activities and should be supported by university leadership.

3. Finally, there is no substitute for mentorship. Integrating health advocacy into a career, no matter what the practice setting, can often seem like uncharted territory. Seeking out mentors who have followed a similar path, or who have related experiences can provide important guidance and support. Pediatricians may need to look outside their own practice setting for this mentorship and may find that they need several different mentors for different aspects of their professional development. In addition to longer term mentors, learning from others' experiences at conferences or through informational meetings can be similarly valuable.

Building skills and leadership in child health advocacy can improve health outcomes for children and increase professional satisfaction. No matter the practice setting, pediatricians can be effective advocates for child health through leveraging organizational, professional, and community resources and partnerships.

CLINICS CARE POINTS

- Collaborations, partnerships, and engagement with professional medical societies can help the busy pediatrician participate in child health advocacy, irrespective of their practice setting.
- Effective mentorship can help support the child health advocate to navigate through complex issues and promote career development.
- Child health advocates facing hostility or conflictual environments are encouraged to seek advice and support from medical societies, their institutions, and/or their mentors to aid them in navigating these difficult issues when needed.

REFERENCES

1. Earnest MA, Wong SL, Federico SG. Physician advocacy: what is it and how do we do it? Acad Med 2010;85(1):63–7.
2. Zipursky AA. History of pediatric specialties. Pediatr Res 2002;52(5):617.
3. Dodson NA, Talib HJ, Gao Q, et al. Pediatricians as child health advocates: the role of advocacy education. Health Promotion Pract 2021;22(1):13–7.
4. Hughes JG. American academy of pediatrics: the first 50 years. Illinois: American Academy of Pediatrics; 50th Anniversary Commemorative ed edition; 1980. p. 1–4.
5. Leonard MB, Pursley DM, Robinson LA, et al. The importance of trustworthiness: lessons from the COVID-19 pandemic. Pediatr Res 2022;91:482–5.
6. Larkin H. Navigating attacks against health care workers in the COVID-19 era. JAMA 2021;325(18):1822–4.
7. Accreditation Council for Graduate Medical Education. ACGME Common program requirements for graduate medical education in pediatrics. In: Accreditation Council for graduate medical education. 2021. Available at: https://www.acgme.org/What-We-Do/Accreditation/Common-Program-Requirements. Accessed June 13, 2022.
8. Howell BA, Kristal RB, Whitmire LR, et al. A systematic review of advocacy curricula in graduate medical education. J Gen Intern Med 2019;34(11):2592–601.
9. Nerlinger AL, Shah AN, Beck AF, et al. The advocacy portfolio: a standardized tool for documenting physician advocacy. Acad Med 2018;93(6):860–8.
10. Keller D, Chamberlain LJ. Children and the patient protection and affordable care act: opportunities and challenges in an evolving system. Acad Pediatr 2014;14(3):225–33.
11. Counts NZ, Roiland RA, Halfon N. Proposing the ideal alternative payment model for children. JAMA Pediatr 2021;175(7):669–70.
12. Alberti P, Fair M, Skorton DJ. Now is our time to act: why academic medicine must embrace community collaboration as its fourth mission. Acad Med 2021;96(11):1503–6.

13. Yu Z, Moustafa D, Kwak R, et al. Engaging in advocacy during medical training: assessing the impact of a virtual COVID-19 focused state advocacy day. Postgrad Med J 2022;98:365–8.
14. Ramirez M, Bruce JS, Ball AJ, et al. Pediatric departmental level advocacy: addressing COVID-19 and racism. J Pediatr 2021;231:7–9e3.
15. Jeelani R, Lieberman D, Chen SH. Is patient advocacy the solution to physician burnout? Semin Reprod Med 2019;37:246–50.
16. Chamberlain LJ, Wu S, Lewis GL, et al. A multi-institutional medical education collaborative: legislative advocacy training in california pediatric residency programs. Acad Med 2013;88(3):314–21.
17. Chung RJ, Ramirez MR, Best DL, et al. Advocacy and community engagement: perspectives from pediatric department chairs. J Pediatr 2022;248. 6.e3–10.e3.

Advocacy in the Community

Community Engagement
How to Form Authentic Partnerships for Lasting Change

Sara M. Bode, MD[a,b]

KEYWORDS

- Community engagement • Advocacy • Pediatric training

KEY POINTS

- Pediatricians play a critical role in promoting child health through community engagement.
- The AAP Community Pediatrics Training Initiative focuses on training faculty and residents in the skills necessary to work alongside the community in authentic engagement.
- These skills train pediatricians to be effective leaders and advocates through development of community partnerships to impact systems and policy change for children.
- Core skills include community assessment and competence, authentic community engagement, and community action through coalition building.

Pediatricians have been working in the community since the start of our profession. Dr Jacobi, the father of pediatrics, discussed the importance of community engagement and leadership as he worked for system change at the community level. "It is not enough, however, to work at the individual bedside in the hospital. In the near or dim future, the pediatrician is to sit in and control school boards, health departments, and legislatures. He is a legitimate advisor to the judge and jury, and a seat for the physician in the counsels of the republic is what the people have a right to demand."[1,2]

Pediatricians have long played a critical role promoting child health through community engagement, working alongside community members in a multidisciplinary team approach to effect change in systems, environment, or access to services that improve the well-being of children and families. The American Academy of Pediatrics (AAP) defines community pediatrics as "the practice of promoting and integrating the positive social, cultural, and environmental influences on children's health as well as addressing potential negative effects that deter optimal child health and development within a community. Community pediatrics includes the following:

[a] Department of Pediatrics, Ohio State University, 700 Children's Drive, Columbus, OH 43205, USA; [b] Department of Community Wellness, Nationwide Children's Hospital
E-mail address: Sara.bode@nationwidechildrens.org
Twitter: @SaraBodeMD (S.M.B.)

Pediatr Clin N Am 70 (2023) 35–41
https://doi.org/10.1016/j.pcl.2022.09.013
0031-3955/23/© 2022 Elsevier Inc. All rights reserved.

- A perspective that expands the pediatrician's focus from one child to the well-being of all children in the community
- A recognition that family, educational, social, cultural, spiritual, economic, environmental, and political forces affect the health and functioning of children
- A synthesis of clinical practice and public health principles to promote the health of all children within the context of the family, school, and community
- A commitment to collaborate with community partners to advocate for and provide quality services equitably for all children."[3]

However, working alongside the community with authentic engagement and lasting system change requires a skill set that is often not the focus of traditional medical training.

The Community Pediatrics Training Initiative (CPTI) is an AAP initiative that focuses on training pediatricians, both residents and faculty, to be effective leaders and advocates through development of authentic community partnerships to impact systems and policy change for children. CPTI provides faculty development opportunities and resources, advocacy training and curricula, and collaboratives across institutions to accelerate advocacy on behalf of children.

These skills require health providers to work outside of traditional clinical venues, with a broad focus on upstream interventions that can affect the entire population of a community. So how do we begin to develop the needed skills and what are the main components of effective community engagement? The core skills of community engagement include the following: completion of a community assessment, community competence, skills of authentic community engagement, skills for community action, and finally assessment and sustainability.

COMMUNITY ASSESSMENT AND COMPETENCE

What does it mean for pediatricians to develop skills in community assessment? It starts with learning how to identify the community with which you want to engage. Communities can coalesce around many different aspects: geography, certain population characteristics, or even a health condition. Many sectors, including public health, use Geographic Information System (GIS) technologies as an emerging tool used to gather, manage, organize, and conceptualize data around health and wellness. Using GIS technology, data can be spatially organized and analyzed on a map to help users recognize patterns and relationships. This technology has been used to discover important patterns in recent years from cancer incidence, to obesity and food resources, to gun violence patterns.[4,5] As an individual pediatrician, the concept of geomapping with the use of data alongside geography, cultural inhabitants, disease prevalence, and health and social resources is a critical skill that can be used to gain insight into a specific community.

Community assessment includes components of geomapping, with a pediatric health lens, to identify assets and challenges in a community that may affect a child's health and wellness. This assessment can include online data gathering combined with both observational and experiential components.

A thoughtful windshield or walking survey activity can be a useful tool to accomplish an initial community assessment. A windshield or walking survey is a structured observational tool used to help identify the needs and assets within a specific community.[6] The AAP CPTI, through expert consensus, developed a windshield/walking survey activity specifically for pediatric health providers.[7] A thoughtful approach to this activity is key. The goal of this survey is not to promote "poverty tourism" but rather a starting point to use an asset-based approach to gain a deepened understanding of your community's strengths and challenges. This activity includes some prework using on-line resources to better understand the health of children in the community of interest. Once the community of interest is identified, pediatricians can use data to understand the demographics of families who live there, and resources available to them, with an emphasis on factors that may affect their health and well-being. Several online data re-sources exist to gather additional information about a community such as the sociode-mographic and other child health indicators of children and families living in the specified area. Example key resources include the Centers for Disease Control (CDC) Youth Risk Behavior Surveillance System (YRBSS),[8] City-Data,[9] and the Annie E. Casey Foundation Kids Count Data Center.[10] Demographics and child health metrics are avail-able for most communities around the country using these and other resources. The CDC YRBSS can give information on risk behaviors such as substance use (alcohol, to-bacco, vaping, and so on), depression/suicide rates, and sexual and intimate partner violence. City-Data pulls public information from several resources to provide informa-tion on vital statistics such as median household income, median house value and rent, family household size, and demographics. This information can often be obtained at a granular level and provide a neighborhood-level picture of the community. Kids Count Data Center focuses specifically on child health metrics and covers several areas such as employment and income (children living below the federal poverty level, chil-dren in poverty by race/ethnicity, level of public assistance, WIC [the special supple-mental nutrition program for women, infants, and children] enrollment), education (students enrolled in state-funded preschool, young children not in school), and com-munity environment (children living in high areas of poverty, children who have experi-enced at least 2 adverse experiences, children without a vehicle at home). These are just a few examples of the many child health indicators that can be obtained as background with the goal to use this information to reflect on how that informs your overall commu-nity assessment as you complete a structured observation of your chosen community.

The next step is to go and assess the neighborhoods using a windshield/walking survey tool, completing a structured checklist. Components of the CPTI windshield/walking survey include observation of the following categories: housing/zoning, retail services, schools/childcare, places of worship, human services, open spaces, trans-portation, public safety, neighborhood life, and socioeconomic status. This structured tool includes a reflection on what was observed, including assets and challenges for children and families in the community. What are the biggest strengths about living and raising children in this community? What are the biggest challenges?[7]

Community competence takes the overall data and observations to the next level; it includes the ability to identify and describe specific assets, needs, and challenges that impact the health and well-being of children and families in the community assessed, and then to identify possible advocacy opportunities through your windshield survey findings to improve the health and well-being of children and families.

Critical to this assessment process is using a respectful, thoughtful, asset-based approach to these observations with the understanding that this is just the beginning of community engagement work. These skills in community assessment and compe-tence lay the groundwork and baseline knowledge needed to then engage with com-munity members to gain further insight and work alongside your community to effect positive change.

AUTHENTIC COMMUNITY ENGAGEMENT

As a pediatrician, authentic community engagement is critical to providing sustainable change toward improved child health outcomes; this includes an understanding of your role in the community, power sharing, and ensuring a shared partnership where all community members' voices are heard.

The National Institute for Children's Health Quality Executive Project Director Kenn Harris states: "The belief behind community engagement is that the people impacted by the problem have some of the best solutions," "They help us understand how they experience the system, *their lived experience*, and that's not something we can learn anywhere else. When those experiences and their voices become part of the solution—when they're combined with organizational knowledge, resources and expertise—it becomes a pretty amazing partnership that inspires innovative thinking."[11]

This speaks to the core components of authentic community engagement, including establishing relationships, building trust, working with formal and informal leadership, and seeking commitment from community organizations and leaders to create processes for mobilizing the community.[12] Community engagement takes a long-term commitment to work with communities, not for or on behalf of them. Working with communities ensures that the population impacted by the problem is involved in cocreating the solutions using an asset-based approach. The community strengths should be at the center of the work while your role brings tools and resources to develop capacity for the needed change. As a pediatrician, understanding each partner's individual and community role is critical to underscore and ensure shared power with decision making. By establishing longitudinal relationships within the community and listening to members you can build trust, which lays the foundation to support community-led solutions. It is important to know that this requires a long-term commitment from the individual, organizations, and other partners.

COMMUNITY ACTION

Once authentic engagement has been established, with a community coalition built to affect a specific change, the work of community organizing gets started.

There are key leadership practices associated with effective community action: telling stories, building relationships, structuring teams, strategizing, and acting. Telling stories involves working to articulate the story of the community, why it is united, and why we must act to effect change.[13] Again, using the voices of diverse community members, from all types of positions and roles, can ensure this story reflects the true lived experience of the community and includes broad inclusive ideas for solutions. Then comes building intentional relationships and structuring a team that distributes both power and responsibility.[13] Strategizing involves cataloguing your resources and linking them to achieve clear goals toward your intended outcomes. Finally, we act, translating that strategy into effective action over time.

As a pediatrician you may find yourself in several different roles and levels of responsibility depending on the community action being taken. Some might be in an advisory capacity, providing critical information such as health data or available resources. Often pediatricians can share stories of cases they have seen, what has motivated their work, and bear witness to the community's struggle. Other community action might involve a leadership role in advancing the work, including partnering to develop the strategies and goals; this may also include working with your institution or professional organization in an official capacity. Knowing what "hat" you are wearing while working alongside a community is important. Representing your hospital, practice, state AAP Chapter, or other organization carries with it a responsibility to represent those interests alongside the community interests. Regardless of the specific role you are taking, these core principles of community engagement and action still apply.

ASSESSMENT AND SUSTAINABILITY

Once community action is underway, assessment becomes necessary as a tool to both measure the effect of your action and provide feedback to all stakeholders in the work, including community members. Make sure this includes publicly sharing the contributions of your community members and partners when sharing success stories. How did using a community-led approach strengthen the outcomes? Who participated and what community assets and expertise contributed to the success? This measurement of success is a large component of sustainability. Each stakeholder can use the outcomes to build internal support at their institutions and as a communication tool for additional funding. Often a key pediatrician role and skill set is employed here—the ability to take outcomes data and share with key organizations to galvanize additional interest and support.

Working alongside a community to engage in system-level change takes a long-term commitment, development of new skills, and the incorporation of nontraditional pediatrician roles. This engagement is also some of the most rewarding, powerful work one can do as a pediatrician to improve the health of children and families.

CASE STUDY

Observation of elementary students attempting to access private hospital playgrounds.

Problem

Pediatric faculty and residents observed that several elementary-aged children over summer months were attempting to access the locked, restricted, hospital playground facilities next to the outpatient academic medical center; this was noted multiple times over several weeks leading to concerns about available play spaces in the local neighborhood surrounding the clinic. In addition, it was noted that the neighborhood surrounding the hospital did not have accessible sidewalks and in fact crossed an interstate and busy intersection, raising concerns for child safety while walking to the facilities.

These observations led to a group of pediatric residents led by 2 faculty members to conduct a community assessment to further understand the scope of the observed problem. The community was identified to include the catchment area for the local elementary school within 0.2 miles of the outpatient pediatric clinic. Online data evaluation and structured windshield surveys were conducted to assess the area. Some conclusions included a significant lack of accessible green and play space with poor walkability of most neighborhoods due to lack of sidewalks or poor road conditions. A noted asset was the elementary school itself, which included a large playground and green space but was not accessible outside of school hours, including summer. Another observation included limited access to grocery stores, none within walking distance, and several local convenience stations that appeared to be used as a common food purchasing source. One local food mart, Cafecito's, appeared to have a significant community presence and strong engagement.

Solution

Through the results of the community assessment, 2 areas of possible intervention were identified: food resources and open play space. Area community members were engaged including school leadership, students, parents through the local Parent Teacher Association (PTA), and Cafecito's. Focus groups were conducted to engage both parents and students, which were coled by the pediatrician group and school leadership to identify community concerns around these topics with potential resources and identified solutions.

A strong theme quickly emerged around the lack of available programs for elementary-aged children over the summer months. This concern extended to lack of places to play outside as well as needs for a summer feeding program.

A community coalition was formed that included the local children's hospital community engagement office, pediatrician group, school leadership, PTA leadership, and additional parents, student liaisons, owner of Cafecito's and the local YMCA chapter. The coalition's goals included providing a sustainable safe summer experience for children aged 4 to 12 years that included food resources and open play space. A second goal included sustainable parent engagement to include nutrition education and resources.

Outcome

Through funding and community support and collaboration, several programs and interventions were employed. First a summer youth program was opened using existing school grounds, which included active play, new materials, and a summer food program serving more than 100 students. The school site was also used for weekly food distribution for all family and community members. The opening of the summer program included a family night with sponsored partnerships to provide onsite resources for families around insurance coverage, medical and dental home establishment, state benefits, food resources, and more. During the school year, monthly parent education sessions, sponsored by Cafecito's and led by the children's hospital pediatricians and staff, focused on child health and wellness were implemented. This new coalition led to ongoing support and structure with sustainable programming each year.

Lessons Learned

Pediatricians are often witnesses to child health needs through their daily practice; they have a unique role and skill set that can be used to effect lasting system change to improve child health outcomes. Using the skills of initial observation and curiosity, along with community assessment and authentic engagement, pediatricians are key advocates leading alongside the community. Advocacy skills around community assessment, engagement, and action are key strategies that are necessary to specifically target for pediatric faculty and trainees to ensure they learn the necessary skills to be effective in this critical domain.

CLINICS CARE POINTS

- Faculty and residents can access training materials and opportunities to improve their community advocacy skills from the AAP CPTI.
- Pediatricians should use online data resources, such as Kids Count Data Center and YRBSS, to identify assets and challenges in a community that may affect a child's health and wellness.
- Effective community engagement requires core skills and a long-term commitment to work alongside communities for system level change to improve child health.

DISCLOSURE

The author has nothing to disclose.

REFERENCES

1. Earnest MA, Wong SL, Federico SG. Perspective: physician advocacy: what is it and how do we do it? Acad Med 2010;85:6367.
2. Oberg CN. Pediatric advocacy: yesterday, today, and tomorrow. Pediatr 2003; 112(2):406–9.
3. Community pediatrics: navigating the intersection of medicine, public health, and social determinants of children's health. council on community pediatrics. Pediatr 2013;131(3):623–8.
4. Musa GJ, Chiang PH, Sylk T, et al. Use of GIS mapping as a public health tool-from cholera to cancer. Health Serv Insights 2013;6:111–6.
5. Using Geo-mapping Technology to assess Obesity and Food Insecurity in Detroit. Pediatrics 2020;146(1_MeetingAbstract):87–90.
6. Rabinowtiz P. Community assessment, Chapter 3. Assessing community needs and resources, section 21. Windshield and walking surveys. Community Tool Box (ku.edu). Center for Community Health and Development, University of Kansas; 2022.
7. AAP CPTI windshield survey tool for pediatric providers. www.aap.org/cpti. Accessed 2 May 2022.
8. Centers for Disease Control (CDC). Youth risk behavior surveillance system. https://www.cdc.gov/healthyyouth/data/yrbs/index.htm. Accessed 2 May 2022.
9. City-Data. https://www.city-data.com/. Accessed 2 May 2022.
10. The Annie E. Casey Foundation Kids Count Data Center. https://datacenter.kidscount.org/. Accessed 2 May 2022.
11. Roadmap for authentic community engagement. National Institute for Children's Health Quality. 2022. https://www.nichq.org/insight/roadmap-authentic-community-engagement. Accessed 2 May 2022.
12. Principles of authentic community engagement. Minnesota Department of Health Center for Public Health Practice, Principles of Authentic Community Engagement (state.mn.us). 2018. Available at: https://www.health.state.mn.us/communities/practice/resources/phqitoolbox/authenticprinciples.
13. Principles of community engagement. 2nd Edition. Centers for Disease Control; 2011. NIH Publication No. 11-7782.

Community Advocacy in Pediatric Practice

Perspectives from the Field

Karen Camero, MD[a], Joyce R. Javier, MD, MPH, MS[b,c],*

KEYWORDS

- Community advocacy • Health equity • Medical education
- Community-based participatory research

KEY POINTS

- Through community advocacy, pediatricians and other child advocates can collaborate with communities to address environmental and social factors that influence child health.
- Pediatric residents are required by the Accreditation Council for Graduate Medical Education to complete ambulatory experiences in community pediatrics and child advocacy, and exposure to these principles increases pediatricians' involvement in community engagement after training.
- Because advocacy curricula are heterogeneous across GME, educational collaboratives can help disseminate information between institutions and engage with community partners.
- General academic pediatric fellowships, involvement with professional societies such as the American Academy of Pediatrics, Academic Pediatrics Association, and Society for Pediatric Research, and participation in coaching/mentorship programs offer opportunities to strengthen advocacy skills and engagement after residency training.
- Community-based participatory research can promote child health equity in minority populations by listening to these communities and helping develop culturally congruent solutions to their problems.
- Community advocacy can play an important role in promoting job satisfaction and preventing moral injury.

Pediatrics is a specialty that is grounded in advocacy, possibly more than any other field of medicine.[1] In fact, the American Academy of Pediatrics (AAP) was founded after the American Medical Association failed to endorse legislation to protect maternal and child health.[1] Perhaps, it is because pediatricians carry the voices of those with

a Children's Hospital Los Angeles; b Department of Pediatrics, Division of General Pediatrics; c Department of Population and Public Health Sciences, Children's Hospital Los Angeles, Keck School of Medicine of the University of Southern California
* Corresponding author. 4650 Sunset Boulevard MS #76, Los Angeles, CA 90027.
E-mail address: JoJavier@chla.usc.edu

Pediatr Clin N Am 70 (2023) 43–51
https://doi.org/10.1016/j.pcl.2022.09.009
0031-3955/23/© 2022 Elsevier Inc. All rights reserved.

little political expression, who cannot advocate for themselves. Infants, children, and adolescents depend on others to cover their basic needs including food, shelter, and education and rely on proxy voices to speak out on their behalf.[2] In this article, we describe the importance of community advocacy in pediatrics, best practices for training pediatricians in community advocacy, and case studies to highlight trainee experiences and demonstrate how community advocacy and community-based participatory research (CBPR) can be incorporated in the career of a pediatrician. We conclude the article with a discussion of how community advocacy can boost the well-being of the pediatric workforce.

IMPORTANCE OF COMMUNITY ADVOCACY

Community advocacy has been an essential part of pediatrics since its inception[3] and today more than ever remains a crucial practice for promoting the well-being of infants, children, and adolescents. According to the AAP, "community advocacy takes into consideration the environmental and social factors influencing child health, such as exposure to violence, safe places to play, poverty, child abuse, and access to healthy foods, and addresses ways in which child advocates—including pediatricians—can work with community partners to address these issues."[4] In addition to collaborating with communities, pediatricians can use their expertise to educate local, state, and national legislators to prioritize and support policies that can improve child health.[3]

The Accreditation Council for Graduate Medical Education has formally included advocacy in the common program requirements for pediatric residency programs, stating that residents should complete ambulatory experiences that include elements of community pediatrics and child advocacy.[5] In response, medical schools, residency programs, and academic health centers are increasingly incorporating curricular units and experiences that encompass social determinants of health, community-based education, and political action.[6]

Residency training provides a unique opportunity for teaching the principles and establishing the practice of community pediatrics[7] because research has shown that exposure to these principles during residency increases pediatricians' involvement in community engagement after training.[8] However, advocacy curricula are heterogeneous across graduate medical education[1] and engagement in advocacy activities during residency is challenging due to barriers such as time constraints and insufficient resources. At a time when stories about racial injustice, mass shootings, threats to reproductive rights, and a mental health crisis dominate US news, we must collaborate to overcome these barriers and prioritize training the next generation of pediatric leaders to become child advocates.

BEST PRACTICES FOR TRAINING PEDIATRICIANS IN COMMUNITY ADVOCACY

Educational collaboratives offer a unique approach to disseminating information between institutions and engaging with community partners. An example of this is the California Collaborative in Community Pediatrics and Legislative Advocacy.[6] This collaborative was founded in 2008 and united 13 pediatric training programs in California with the goal of strengthening curricula in community pediatrics and legislative advocacy training and has resulted in an increase in advocacy activities across the state.[6] Many pediatric residencies in the nation also have specific tracks that focus on community pediatrics and advocacy. Children's Hospital Los Angeles (CHLA) offers a longitudinal community health and advocacy experience, through a dedicated track called Improving Medicine: Pediatricians and Communities Together, or IMPACT. This program is designed for pediatric residents who desire an in-depth experience involving community-based intervention or policy work.[9] Participants are assigned a mentor and have dedicated time during all 3 years of residency to work on developing and implementing a project.[9] At the end of the project period, residents evaluate their project in a research framework and present their findings at an academic meeting and the hospital's grand rounds.[9] Residents in the IMPACT program also have the opportunity to travel to Sacramento to advocate at the state level with the American Academy of Pediatrics California Chapters.

Beyond residency training, many opportunities exist regarding how to get involved with community advocacy and find mentoring opportunities. First, fellowship training in general academic pediatrics, health services such as the RWJF Faculty Scholars and Clinical Scholars Programs, and other pediatric subspecialities is one avenue to continue community advocacy under the mentorship of senior mentors in the field. Second, becoming involved in pediatric academic societies such as the AAP, APA, and Society for Pediatric Research (SPR) can open the doors to advocacy opportunities for pediatricians. For example, one can get involved with their AAP State Chapters or committees such as the Council on Community Pediatrics, Council on Federal Government Affairs, or any of the numerous councils. SPR has an Advocacy Committee that encourages junior members to get involved and also works with the Pediatric Policy Council to advocate for policies that promote child health. The AAP also provides advising to assist in writing Op-Eds and testifying in government settings. The APA also offers the Health Policy Scholars Program, a new 3-year faculty development program designed to help members develop a systematic and scholarly approach to health policy and advocacy. Finally, pediatricians can get involved with local legislators, community leaders through involvement with school boards, PTA, city council, and local public health departments. Many academic institutions are working on creating and implementing coaching programs as avenues to build peer support networks and improve physician wellness. These programs can capture trainees as early as medical school or residency, and extend to fellows and junior faculty members, and can be an innovative approach to plant the advocacy seed into future generations.

CASE STUDY: TRAINEE EXPERIENCES IN THE COMMUNITY

In this next section, we describe the community advocacy experiences of a previous CHLA pediatric residency graduate and current General Academic Pediatric fellow, Dr Karen Camero.

Dr Camero culminated her pediatric residency as COVID-19 was making its debut and leaving many of her patients struggling in various ways, including financially. Although the clinic provided information and resources for households with food insecurity, families were having difficulty paying for other essential products that were not available in food pantries or school meal drives—goods such as diapers or gasoline to fuel their vehicles. Acknowledging the pandemic's financial impact on so many families, the CHLA residency program's Diversity and Inclusion Committee, led by Dr Camero organized an initiative to collect money for the purchase of gift cards. This activity was repeated several times throughout the year and accomplished the creation of a gift card bank that clinic providers could use to distribute cash cards to families in need. The CHLA residency program's Diversity and Inclusion Committee is a group where residents, fellows, and faculty members can come together to support each other and expand cultural awareness and sensitivity.[10] Social responsibility is a core value of this group because it maintains a commitment to the surrounding community by addressing barriers to care for children and empowering patients and their families to improve health.[10]

In addition to community engagement, legislative advocacy was also reinforced through Dr Camero's pediatric training. During her first week at CHLA, she was photographed alongside other first-year pediatric residents while holding up signs that read "Protect Children's Health Care NOW." Later that day, the image would be posted on social media, with the hashtag #keepkidscovered. Dr Susan Wu, a CHLA pediatrician and member of the California Collaborative in Community Pediatrics and Legislative Advocacy, accompanied by other faculty leaders were advocating for the reauthorization of the Children's Health Insurance Program, which became threatened in the year 2017. That same year, Dr Camero and the whole pediatric intern class had the opportunity to visit local legislators to discuss bills supported by the AAP. The CHLA residency program organizes this activity annually with every new cohort of pediatric interns, and pediatric faculty accompanies them during these visits. This activity began as a direct result of the California Collaborative in Community Pediatrics and Legislative Advocacy emphasis described earlier in this article. Training at a hospital that serves a vulnerable patient population gives residents the opportunity to collect many impactful stories to share with their local representatives. Stories that highlight the importance of supporting bills in favor of affordable childcare, gun control, school meal programs, tobacco product regulation and many other topics pertinent to child and adolescent health.

Dr Camero's introduction to advocacy during residency boosted her desire to work closely with the LatinX community in the Los Angeles area and led her to pursue a general academic pediatric fellowship with a focus on health equity, at CHLA. General academic pediatrics fellowships are focused on developing trainees' academic skills in research, advocacy, and medical education scholarship.[11] Academic generalists have important roles in educating medical students and residents. Their research covers significant pediatric topics and informs health policy and program development in ways that improve child and adolescent health.[12] The Pediatrics Fellowship in Health Equity at CHLAs is a 2-year, with an optional third year program that aims to train future leaders in providing high-quality care to all children with a focus on the underserved.[13]

Dr Camero began her pediatric health equity fellowship in the year 2020, which marked a pivotal year in world history. In March of 2020, the World Health Organization declared COVID-19 a pandemic. It was also a year scheduled for presidential elections in the United States. These 2 major events motivated Dr Camero to stay up to date with the latest news because of the influence it had on her patients, their families, and their communities. She was determined to disseminate educational information on social media to counteract misinformation circulating in the Spanish speaking communities during this period, especially about COVID-19 immunizations. Thanks to the protected educational time and mentorship awarded by the fellowship, she was able to work on various projects focused on addressing health disparities. One example was the implementation of an anticipatory guidance passport in the pediatric continuity clinic, which focused on increasing the skills of first-year pediatric residents in providing patient oriented and culturally sensitive counseling on topics such as parenting, nutrition, and social determinants of health. Through a series of structured lectures and meetings with community partners, she grew more aware of the needs of her community and the efforts already in existence aimed at addressing them. Dr Camero's main research project, as discussed in future sections of this article, involved the implementation and evaluation of positive parenting workshops delivered to Spanish-speaking mothers of infants. Altogether, this fellowship allowed Dr Camero to better appreciate the importance of community advocacy and gave her the framework, tools, and mentorship to continue her work in this area. This job has been extremely fulfilling to her and she advises general academic pediatric programs to better advertise their existence, so current pediatric residents become aware of this option as a pipeline for a career in academic medicine, where they can later help shape future pediatric advocates.

CASE STUDY DESCRIBING FACULTY EXPERIENCES

The Filipino Family Health Initiative (FFHI)[14] is an example of an over-decade-long community advocacy research partnership that involves pediatric academic partners and community-based organizations. In a later section of this article, we share the story behind the origins of FFHI to highlight 3 important points: (1) the importance of giving physicians in training early exposure to community advocacy and CBPR, (2) lessons learned from incorporating advocacy and CBPR in a pediatrician's career, and (3) how community advocacy can lead to innovative, culturally congruent methods to promote child health equity.

EXPOSING PHYSICIANS-IN-TRAINING TO ADVOCACY AND COMMUNITY-BASED PARTICIPATORY RESEARCH

The Community Advocacy Rotation, previously called STAT at the Stanford Pediatric Residency Program at Lucile Packard Children's Hospital was the senior author's first exposure to how to incorporate community advocacy in a pediatrician's career. Under the mentorship of Dr Lisa Chamberlain, Dr Javier partnered with community-based organizations serving Filipino youth to tackle the problem of teen pregnancy using principles of community-based participatory research. She was able to obtain an American Academy of Pediatrics Community Access to Child Health Grant to fund this study and published her findings in a peer-reviewed journal.[15]

This project involved partnering with a community-based organization called the Filipino Youth Coalition in Milpitas, CA. Together, we organized a campaign regarding how to prevent teen pregnancy, which culminated in 2 parent–teen conferences. These conferences included conversations about how to bridge the communication gap between first-generation Filipino parents and their second-generation children growing up in the United States, as well as tips for parents on how to talk about sex with your teen. A major outcome from the first conference was the securing of funding from a private foundation for a second conference. Qualitative feedback from a postsurvey evaluation revealed that the community appreciated the cultural tailoring of this event.

As part of this project, Dr Javier also asked youth who attended the parent–teen conference: what are the most dangerous issues affecting them today? The youth's answer was mental and emotional health. Listening to the youth's voices, Dr Javier decided to focus future advocacy efforts on promoting the emotional well-being of youth in the Filipino community. She also learned from community leaders about the power of data and the need to increase the collection of disaggregated data in the Asian American, Native Hawaiian and Pacific Islander communities so that community-based organizations can advocate for the health needs of specific AANHPI subgroups, such as Filipino Americans. This discovery and mentored experiences during residency led her to pursue a postdoctoral fellowship in general academic pediatrics and Masters of Public Health degree in Epidemiology.

Lessons Learned from Incorporating Advocacy and community-based participatory research in a Pediatrician's Career

Dr Javier learned several lessons from using community-based participatory research and community advocacy in her career. First, she learned the importance of listening to the community, and building on its strengths in order to develop culturally congruent solutions to wicked problems, such as adolescent behavioral health disparities. Building on the skills she learned as a resident, the first step to determining how to prevent adolescent behavioral health problems among Filipino youth was to ask the community: What are the mental health issues affecting Filipino teens and what can we do to prevent them? She conducted a mixed-methods study and interviewed adolescents, grandparents, parents, teachers, health and mental health providers, clergy, and local government leaders. Their collective answer was to not wait until they are adolescents but to focus on the school-age years and promote stronger parent–child relationships by offering the Incredible Years, an evidence-based parenting intervention in churches.[16–18] Second, she learned the importance of building on the strengths of Filipino cultural values while balancing the importance of raising awareness about stigmatized issues such as suicide and depression in this community. This delicate balance is evident in a culturally tailored and theory-based video[19] that was developed by a parent community advisory board and aimed at increasing enrollment rates in evidence-based parenting workshops.[20] Filipino parents demonstrated the cultural values of *kapwa* (shared identity) and *bayanihan* (giving to others without expecting anything in return, or communal unity) by sharing testimonials as to why they enrolled in the incredible years and the benefits of the program on their relationships with their children. These parents also encouraged Dr Javier to include statistics about Filipino behavioral health disparities in the video as this may increase a parent's perceived susceptibility that their child may be at risk for adolescent risky behaviors such as substance abuse and suicidal behavior. This video was evaluated in a randomized controlled trial and was found to be effective in increasing enrollment rates in parenting workshops.[21]

How Community Advocacy can Promote Child Health Equity

Compared with other race/ethnicities, Filipino adolescents have higher rates of suicidal behavior.[22] The FFHI has been working to prevent and address Filipino adolescent health disparities for over a decade. Part of this study also involved a campaign to create a culture of mental health and healthy parenting in the Filipino community using funding from the Robert Wood Johnson Foundation's Clinical Scholar's program. This campaign began by focusing on how to make mental health a shared value by conducting focus groups with Filipino stakeholders in order to create a shared definition of adolescent mental health for and by the community. This definition was shared in a conference aimed at decreasing mental health stigma in the community, and lessons learned from offering positive parenting programs in the Filipino community were also shared. To date more than 175 families have participated in evidence-based parenting workshops aimed at improving parent–child relationships and communication during the school-age years. Outcomes we have seen from evaluations of the program include increased the use of positive parenting strategies such as praise and decreased parenting stress, child internalizing and externalizing symptoms, and child depressive and anxiety symptoms.[16]

FFHI had to adapt during the COVID-19 pandemic. Before the pandemic, we partnered with more than 30 community-based organizations and offered workshops in person to Filipino families living in Southern California. During the COVID-19 pandemic, we transitioned to online implementation,[23] which enabled us to offer workshops statewide in California and engage additional community partners in the San Francisco Bay area, Davis and in Stockton. We were also able to obtain funding to offer workshops in the Philippines and the rest of the United States.

By listening to the community and using principles of community-based participatory research, the FFHI is an example of how community advocacy can promote child health equity in a population often called an invisible minority in the United States. The FFHI has recently expanded to include the LatinX community. During the pandemic, we began reaching out to Spanish-speaking families to increase the outreach of evidence-based parenting workshops among communities of color to address the mental health crisis affecting youth in other minority groups. The second author Dr Karen Camero is leading this effort with Spanish-speaking families under the mentorship of Dr Javier. Overall, using CBPR to advocate for communities has enabled us to increase the participation of minorities in research, a theme also described in a recent 10-year systematic review[24] and a critical step to achieving health equity.

In summary, this article shares the importance of community advocacy in pediatrics and demonstrates the importance of using principles of community-based participatory research when defining needs, priorities, strengths, and solutions. A last take home message to emphasize would be the role community advocacy plays in promoting job satisfaction and preventing moral injury, a term referring to a provider's inability to provide high-quality care due to the systems and culture of health care surrounding the provider.[25] Being involved with community advocacy helps pediatricians return to the reasons why they pursued a career in medicine and think like an active agent and partner in driving systemic change to improve health for all communities, regardless of their background. Given the recent mass shootings and mental health crisis, and continued presence of racism and discrimination in the United States, more than ever, we need to preserve the well-being of the pediatric workforce so that they can continue to advocate for the youth of this nation.

CLINICS CARE POINTS

- Pediatricians should not wait to be experts in advocacy before participating in advocacy activities. As child health experts, pediatricians carry the voices of their patients and families, which is very valuable for the advocacy process.

- Pediatricians who engage in community advocacy need to avoid working in isolation and, instead, partner with other child advocates and community leaders to advance child health.[26]

- Pediatricians should not feel obligated to engage in numerous advocacy activities but rather align their advocacy efforts with their interests because research suggests that physicians who engage in the work that they find most meaningful are at significantly lower risk of burnout.[25]

- When conducting community-based participatory research, pediatric professionals must collaborate with community members on all aspects of the project, including needs assessment, planning, design, implementation, evaluation, and dissemination.[27]

ACKNOWLEDGMENTS

Joyce Javier has received funding from the Robert Wood Johnson Foundation, USC Keck School of Medicine Bridge Funds & COVID-19 Research Fund. This research was also funded by grant K23HD071942 from the Eunice Kennedy Shriver National Institute for Child Health and Human Development, grants UL1TR001855 and UL1TR000130 from the National Center for Advancing Translational Science of the US National Institutes of Health, and Community Access to Child Health (CATCH) grants from the American Academy of Pediatrics. The content is solely the responsibility of the authors and does not necessarily represent the official views of the National Institutes of Health, RWJF, USC, or AAP.

REFERENCES

1. Dodson NA, Talib HJ, Gao Q, et al. Pediatricians as child health advocates: the role of advocacy education. Health Promotion Pract 2021;22(1):13–7.
2. Oberg CN. Pediatric advocacy: yesterday, today, and tomorrow. Pediatrics (Evanston) 2003;112(2):406–9.
3. Shah SI, Brumberg HL. Advocating for advocacy in pediatrics: supporting life-long career trajectories. Pediatrics (Evanston) 2014;134(6):e1523–7.
4. American Academy of Pediatrics. Learn about community advocacy. 2021. Available at: https://www.aap.org/en/advocacy/community-health-and-advocacy/learn-about-community-advocacy/. Accessed June 5, 2022.
5. Accreditation Council for Graduate Medical Education. Program requirements for residency education in pediatrics. Available at: https://www.acgme.org/globalassets/PFAssets/ProgramRequirements/320_Pediatrics_2020.pdf?ver=2020-06-29-162726-647&ver=2020-06-29-162726-647. Accessed May 20, 2022.
6. Chamberlain LJ, Wu S, Lewis G, et al. A multi-institutional medical educational collaborative: advocacy training in California pediatric residency programs. Acad Med 2013;88(3):314–21.
7. Shipley LJ, Stelzner SM, Zenni EA, et al. Teaching community pediatrics to pediatric residents: strategic approaches and successful models for education in community health and child advocacy. Pediatrics (Evanston) 2005;115(4): 1150–7.
8. Lichtenstein C, Hoffman BD, Moon RY. How do US pediatric residency programs teach and evaluate community pediatrics and advocacy training? Acad Pediatr 2017;17(5):544–9.
9. Children's hospital Los Angeles, IMPACT program. Available at: https://www.chla.org/impact-program. Accessed June 2, 2022.
10. Children's Hospital Los Angeles. Diversity and inclusion committee. Available at: https://www.chla.org/diversity-and-inclusion-committee. Accessed June 20, 2022.
11. Academic Pediatric Association. Overview of fellowship programs. Available at: https://www.academicpeds.org/publications-resources/fellowships/overview-of-fellowship-programs/. Accessed June 2, 2022.
12. Council of Pediatric Subspecialties. Academic generalist. Available at: https://www.pedsubs.org/about-cops/subspecialty-descriptions/academic-generalist/. Accessed June 2, 2022.
13. Children's Hospital Los Angeles. Pediatrics fellowship in health equity. Available at: https://www.chla.org/fellowship/pediatrics-fellowship-health-equity. Accessed June 2, 2022.
14. Sepulveda A, David J, Coffey DM, et al. Toolkit for prevention of behavioral health disparities in an immigrant community. 2019. https://img1.wsimg.com/blobby/go/6b6576a4-a4ac-4c32-8b74-0fa6b3fdbc0d/downloads/TOOLKIT-.PDF?ver=1579202031316. Accessed June 15 2022.
15. Javier JR, Chamberlain LJ, Rivera KK, et al. Lessons learned from a community-academic partnership addressing adolescent pregnancy prevention in filipino american families. Prog Community Health Partnerships 2010;4(4):305–13.

16. Javier JR, Coffey DM, Schrager SM, et al. Parenting intervention for prevention of behavioral problems in elementary school-age filipino-american children: a pilot study in churches. J Dev Behav Pediatr 2016;37(9):737–45.
17. Javier JR, Supan J, Lansang A, et al. Preventing filipino mental health disparities: perspectives from adolescents, caregivers, providers, and advocates. Asian Am J Psychol 2014;5(4):316–24.
18. Javier JR, Galura K, Aliganga FAP, et al. Voices of the filipino community describing the importance of family in understanding adolescent behavioral health needs. Fam Community Health 2018;41(1):64–71.
19. Javier JR. The use of an educational video to increase suicide awareness and enrollment in parenting interventions among filipinos. Asian Am J Psychol 2018; 9(4):327–33.
20. Flores N, Supan J, Kreutzer CB, et al. Prevention of Filipino youth behavioral health disparities: Identifying barriers and facilitators to participating in "incredible years," an evidence-based parenting intervention, Los Angeles, California, 2012. Preventing Chronic Dis 2015;12(10):E178.
21. Javier JR, Coffey DM, Palinkas LA, et al. Promoting enrollment in parenting programs among a Filipino population: A randomized trial. Pediatrics (Evanston) 2019;143(2):1.
22. Javier JR, Huffman LC, Mendoza FS. Filipino child health in the United States: do health and health care disparities exist? Preventing Chronic Dis 2007;4(2):A36.
23. Macam SR, Mack W, Palinkas L, et al. Evaluating an evidence-based parenting intervention among filipino parents: protocol for a pilot randomized controlled trial. JMIR Res Protoc 2022;11(2):e21867.
24. Julian McFarlane S, Occa A, Peng W, et al. Community-based participatory research (CBPR) to enhance participation of racial/ethnic minorities in clinical trials: a 10-year systematic review. Health Commun 2021;1–18. https://doi.org/10.1080/10410236.2021.1943978.
25. Dilley K, Javier JR. As we work to boost doctors' well-being, let's retire the term 'burnout'. American Academy of Pediatrics Voices Blog. Available at: https://www.aap.org/en/news-room/aap-voices/as-we-work-to-boost-doctors-well-being-lets-retire-the-term-burnout/. Accessed May 20, 2021.
26. American Academy of Pediatrics. Advocacy guide: effective advocacy at the community, state and federal levels. Available at. www.aap.org/moc/advocacyguide. Accessed September 2, 2022.
27. National Institute on Minority Health and Health Disparities. Community-based participatory research program. 2018. Available at. https://www.nimhd.nih.gov/programs/extramural/community-based-participatory.html. Accessed September 2, 2022.

Advocacy on the State Level

Making Maternal Child Health a Population Health Priority in Maryland

Tina L. Cheng, MD, MPH[a,b]

KEYWORDS

- Maternal • Child health • Medicaid • Advocacy • Legislation • Politics • State
- Health policy

KEY POINTS

- State legislative advocacy can be an effective means to strengthen maternal child health.
- Stories about children and families are powerful. Coupled with a clear message for specific actions can produce empathy and outrage, clarify facts, and help persuade.
- Building relationships with other advocates, community leaders, and legislators can catalyze advocacy efforts.
- Dissemination of the message takes purposeful effort, involves multiple modalities and target audiences, and requires persistence.

Characteristics of Strong Leaders and Advocates: the T's

Tough-minded

Thick-skinned

Tenacious

Tender-hearted

Catherine DeAngelis, MD

Pediatrician Paul Wise has said that pediatric clinicians are "the ultimate witnesses to failed social policy." We have many stories illustrating the need for stronger protections for children, adolescents, and families and for child advocacy. In my previous role as Chair of Pediatrics at Johns Hopkins University and Pediatrician-In-Chief of

---

[a] Department of Pediatrics, University of Cincinnati College of Medicine, Cincinnati, OH, USA;
[b] Cincinnati Children's Hospital Medical Center, 3333 Burnet Avenue MLC 3016, Cincinnati, OH 45229, USA
E-mail address: Tina.Cheng@cchmc.org

Pediatr Clin N Am 70 (2023) 53–65
https://doi.org/10.1016/j.pcl.2022.09.010
pediatric.theclinics.com
0031-3955/23/© 2022 Elsevier Inc. All rights reserved.

the Johns Hopkins Children's Center, I felt a responsibility to serve as chief advocate for children, adolescents, and families in my institution, city, state, and beyond. Our tripartite mission included clinical care, education, and research—but to fully realize our vision to create "the future of child health," advocacy was the necessary fourth leg of the stool. This article presents a case study of how advocacy at the state level led to 2 significant outcomes: maternal child health (MCH) named as one of the 3 Maryland population-health priorities, and the governor launching a US$72 million Maternal and Child Health Care Initiative. Key lessons learned are described.

Children are our most precious asset. Although children aged younger than 18 years make up 24% of the US population, they are the focus of only 9% of the federal budget.[1] US health care spending on children aged younger than 20 years constitutes 10.7% of the overall budget.[2] Public spending on children and families as a percentage of gross domestic product (GDP) is much higher in other industrialized countries compared with the United States, and this spending is correlated with child health outcomes.[3] Although children are a small percentage of the US budget, they are 100% of our future. Ensuring their well-being, for their own sake, and as an investment in the future, is our utmost responsibility.

Unfortunately, children do not vote and a higher proportion of American children than adults live in poverty.[3] Investment in children, adolescents, and families and in disadvantaged populations has been proven to yield improved health outcomes and cost savings.[3–5] Yet, since adults impose the largest cost on the health-care system, many population health efforts have focused on high-cost adults and the Medicare population, with less attention to prevention and the MCH population.

The Academic Pediatric Association has described a 4-step approach to advocacy, which is used to frame this Maryland case study:

1. Identify the issue and target audience,
2. Craft the message,
3. Develop relationships and coalitions, and
4. Communicate the message.

STEP 1: IDENTIFY THE ISSUE AND TARGET AUDIENCE

The state of Maryland has a unique all-payer rate-setting system for hospital services. The model developed by the state and Centers for Medicare and Medicaid Services (CMS) approved in January 2014 shifts from volume-based reimbursement to a global budget revenue system, in an effort to align hospital incentives with community and primary care efforts. Overseen by the Maryland Department of Health and the Maryland Health Services Cost Review Commission (HSCRC), the Total Cost of Care Model incentivizes hospitals to support population health. Because children contribute only a small portion of the total cost in the health-care system, initial population health efforts focused on Medicare and adults.

Initial areas of state priority were diabetes, opioid use, and establishment of the Maryland Primary Care Program. Despite clear roots of many health conditions in childhood, emphasis was on adults. The Maryland Primary Care Program offered prospective payments for advanced primary care but eligibility was based on a minimum number of Medicare beneficiaries. Very few in the MCH population are insured by Medicare and thus MCH practices are not included. Although it is well known that obesity contributes to the development of diabetes and that childhood obesity is strongly linked to adult obesity, state efforts focused on adults.[6] Similarly, it is known that 90% of Americans who meet the clinical criteria for addiction started using substances before the age of 18 years.[7] Primary prevention activities were not included in the state plan. Longer term prevention and MCH were not a priority.

Health-care delivery systems followed the state's lead in their investments. With pediatrics and obstetrics part of large health-care delivery systems under global budgeting, the focus was on the majority adult population and Medicare metrics. Attention in Medicaid focused on dual-eligible beneficiaries who receive both Medicare and Medicaid—in other words, adults.

Although adult health needs dominate medical costs and poor health outcomes, growing evidence spotlights opportunities to address the early conditions that cause individuals to become high-cost, high-need patients in the first place. The record shows that the path to becoming a high-risk, high-needs adult starts as early as in utero and infancy, and that conditions during childhood greatly affect individual health trajectories across the life course. Thus, bending the cost curve and improving health outcomes is a powerful win-win opportunity. However, doing so demands a focus on upstream factors and efforts to eliminate racial/ethnic and socioeconomic disparities.

Thus, the core issue was to strengthen MCH as an effective and efficient way to address those upstream factors. Return on investment has been demonstrated but requires longer term societal investment and advocacy. The target audience was state and federal policymakers.

STEP 2: CRAFT THE MESSAGE

A good message states the problem and why it matters. It must capture and sustain the attention of the target audience. It gives the big picture by providing context, underscoring why it matters now, and creating a sense of urgency. A strong message will also offer a clear demand for specific actions. Stories about children and families are powerful and have broad appeal. Well-told stories can produce empathy and outrage, explain facts, and help persuade. In influencing decision-makers, it is important to personalize communication, include a direct appeal, and communicate more than once (**Box 1**).

In Maryland, crafting the message involved explaining the urgent health needs of children and families, describing why investing in children is critical for our future, discussing demonstrated return on investment, and delivering the message to those who can help. The Coronavirus Disease 2019 (COVID-19) pandemic added urgency to the need to focus on MCH. Some of our specific messaging is seen in **Box 2**.

As leader of a children's hospital and a major provider of pediatric services, I partnered with pediatric leaders at other hospitals and primary care clinicians through the

---

Box 1
Influencing Decision-makers, AmericanAcademy of Pediatrics Advocacy Guide, 2009, p. 58[8]

- *Make Your Communication Personal*: Tell your story and help put a real face on your issue. Let your decision-maker know how your issue directly affects their constituents or community members

- *Include a Direct Appeal*: It is important to include a concrete request from your decision-maker. Be clear about what they can do to support your issue, whether it is their leadership, their vote, or another form of support

- *Communicate More than Once:* Do not be afraid to initiate ongoing or repeated contact with your decision-maker. The more they hear from you, the more they will get to know your issue (and eventually you) and be inspired to act.

Box 2
Crafting the Message on Maternal Child Health from Maryland Bill (HB520/SB406)

There is an urgent need to invest early in the lives of Marylanders to improve the overall and long-term health of the State and ensure health equity. The COVID-19 pandemic has worsened family stress, child hunger, poverty, and child and adolescent mental health globally and in our state and has exposed huge inequities by race/ethnicity.[11–13] In 2018, 12% of Maryland children lived in poverty with great racial/ethnic disparity. This was concentrated in certain regions, such as Baltimore city, where more than 1 in 4 children live in poverty.[14] Poverty rates in Maryland and in the nation are highest among children.[15] Past recessions, similar to the one we are experiencing, have often affected children the most, and they have experienced the longest consequences.[13,16,17] Forecasting estimates of poverty during the COVID-19 crisis suggest that poverty rates in the United States could reach their highest levels in more than 50 years, with working-age adults and children facing particularly large increases. The poverty rate for children is projected to increase by 53%.[13]

According to the Centers for Disease Control and Prevention, Maryland's maternal mortality rate from 2013 to 2017 (24.8 maternal deaths per 100,000 live births) ranks 22nd among all states. The maternal mortality rate for African Americans is almost 4 times that of whites (44.7 maternal deaths vs 11.3 per 100,000 live births).[18,19] For infant and neonatal mortality, Maryland ranks 35th and 39th among the states, respectively. These mortalities are significantly higher than the national rate.[20] Before the pandemic, rates of mental, emotional, and behavioral disorders, including depression, suicide, anxiety, and self-harm, were increasing among children and youth.[21,22] For the 2017 birth cohort, the financial toll of untreated perinatal mood and anxiety disorders is projected to cost US$14 billion, from conception to 5 years postpartum.[23] Healthy People 2020 goals on maternal, infant, and child health (MCH) focus on improving the health and well-being of women, infants, children, and families.[24] Sentinel MCH health indicators require Statewide and national attention.

MCH forms the foundation for health across the life span through adulthood. The MCH population includes women, children, adolescents, and families. Addressing family contextual factors, social needs, and early manifestations of physical and behavioral health conditions in the preconception, prenatal, child, and adolescent stages of life will produce long-term improvements in population health and will strengthen the economic sustainability of Maryland's health systems. A growing body of research demonstrates that adult chronic diseases originate early in the life course, illustrating the need for preventive strategies.[25–27]

Prevention also saves money. The incremental lifetime medical cost of an obese 10-year-old child relative to a child who maintains a healthy weight through adulthood is US$19,000. Multiplying this by the number of obese 10-year-olds today yields a total direct medical cost of obesity of US$14 billion for this age alone.[28] Children are our greatest resource and are the message we send to the future. Making sure they are born healthy, ready to learn, and on a trajectory to healthy adulthood must be our highest priority.

Maryland American Academy of Pediatric chapter. I met with leaders in our state and local departments of health to partner on initiatives. These leaders included the state Medicaid and MCH directors, Medicaid managed care organization directors, Maryland HSCRC, and state and local leaders on maternal and child health and population health. Routinely, we invited legislators to visit our hospital and clinics to discuss the needs of children, adolescents, and families in our community and to highlight the important work being done. In this way, I was fortunate to meet my state senator, Bill Ferguson, a former Teach for America school teacher and attorney, and recognized our shared interest in child and family well-being. A few weeks after that visit to our hospital, we met again at a community event and had further discussion on

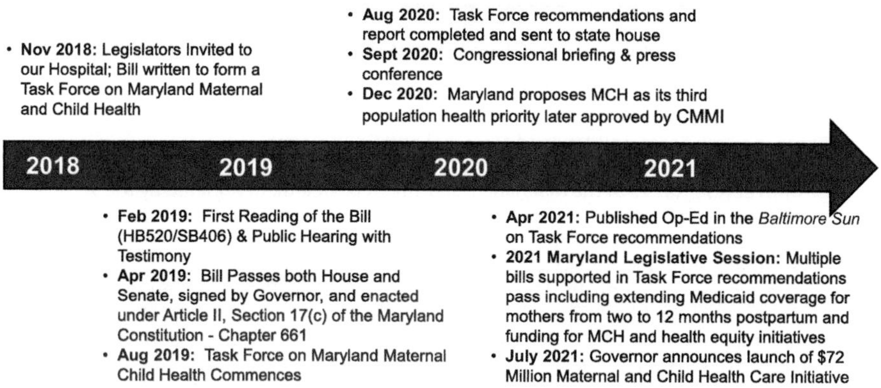

Fig. 1. Timeline of Maryland Legislation Elevating Maternal Child Health starting with House Bill 520/Senate Bill 406.

the challenges facing children and families, especially those on Medicaid, and the difficulty getting attention to these issues in our state and health-care delivery system. He expressed concern and mentioned a bill he would be reintroducing on care coordination for prenatal and infant care. He offered the opportunity to add something to the bill if I was interested in proposing language. This would be the beginning of a collaborative effort that eventually led to cochairing a state task force, implementing task force recommendations, and supporting additional legislative bills (see timeline, **Fig. 1**).

Although I had limited experience in bill writing, I conferred with colleagues in pediatrics and public health and learned about legislative activities in other states related to upstream prevention in MCH. Building on this advice, language was drafted to establish a Maryland Maternal Child Task Force that would review the impact of the State's All Payer System on maternal child health and opportunities for population health. Specifically, the proposed Task Force would recommend how the HSCRC and Maryland Department of Health could incentivize early intervention to prevent adverse MCH outcomes such as asthma, adverse birth outcomes, sickle cell crisis, and mental health crises. The task force would also examine how state policies and payment mechanisms could support partnerships and collaborations for community-based and school-based models of care and address disparities.

A key component of our message was that a greater commitment to the health of children was essential to improve health and lower costs in Maryland. To support this message, we highlighted evidence-based interventions that clearly demonstrate opportunities to improve outcomes for Maryland's families and children. We emphasized that investment early in the life course would ensure healthier pregnancies, healthier children, and a chance for payers to save money in areas such as high-risk maternity care, long infant neonatal intensive care unit (NICU) stays, and children's ED visits and hospitalizations. It would offer a chance to improve the health of Marylanders for decades to come.

The legislation encouraged Medicaid use of the core set of Children's Health Care Quality Measures to monitor improvements, and the bill included specifics on the membership of the Task Force and deadlines for the completion of the report.

STEP 3: DEVELOP RELATIONSHIPS AND COALITIONS

Developing relationships with decision-makers is key in keeping informed on issues and creating change. Constituency building provides strength in numbers. Getting

---

Box 3

Maryland Bill Language to form a Task Force on Maternal and Child Health (HB520)

AN ACT concerning Prenatal and Infant Care Coordination–Grant Funding and Task Force
SECTION 2. AND BE IT FURTHER ENACTED, That:
a. There is a Task Force on Maryland Maternal and Child Health.
b. The Task Force consists of the following members:
    1. one representative of the Maryland Department of Health, designated by the Secretary of Health;
    2. one representative of the Maryland Department of Human Services, designated by the Secretary of Human Services;
    3. one representative of the Maryland Medical Assistance Program, designated by the Secretary of Health;
    4. one representative of the Health Services Cost Review Commission, designated by the Executive Director of the Commission; and
    5. the following members, appointed by the Secretary of Health:
        i. one representative of Johns Hopkins Children's Center;
        ii. one representative from a community–based organization focused on maternal and infant care support and currently partnered with Johns Hopkins Children's Center;
        iii. one representative of University of Maryland Children's Hospital; (iv) one representative from a community–based organization focused on maternal and infant care support and currently partnered with University of Maryland Children's Hospital; and
        v. three representatives of participants who qualify, are receiving or have received care coordination from targeted programs within the current care coordination system;
        vi. one representative of the Maryland Affiliate of the American College of Nurse Midwives;
        vii. one representative of the Maryland Chapter of the American Academy of Pediatrics;
        viii. one representative of the Maryland Association for the Treatment of Opioid Dependence; and
        ix. one physician specializing in neonatology, maternal fetal medicine, or pediatric cardiology from a hospital other than the Johns Hopkins Children's Center or the University of Maryland Children's Hospital; (x) one representative of the Maryland Patient Safety Center; and
        xi. one representative of the Maryland Section of the American College of Obstetricians and Gynecologists.
c. The Secretary of Health shall designate the Chair of the Task Force.
d. The Maryland Department of Health, Maryland Department of Human Services, and the Health Services Cost Review Commission jointly shall provide staff for the Task Force.
e. A member of the Task Force:
    1. may not receive compensation as a member of the Task Force; but
    2. is entitled to reimbursement for expenses under the Standard State Travel Regulations, as provided in the State budget.
f. The Task Force shall study and make recommendations on:
    1. how the policies of the Health Services Cost Review Commission Maryland Department of Health can be used to incentivize early intervention and prevention of key adverse health outcomes, such as asthma, adverse birth outcomes, sickle cell crisis, and mental health crises; and
    2. how State policies and payment mechanisms can:
        i. support community–based and school–based models of care;
        ii. use the global budgets revenue system encourage partnerships under the all–payer model to improve child care;
        iii. assist in collaborations with public health care; and
        iv. use the Core Set of Children's Health Care Quality Measures for Medicaid to monitor improvements; and
    3. programs that the Maryland Medical Assistance Program should implement.

g. On or before November 1, 2019, the Task Force shall report its findings and recommendations to the General Assembly in accordance with § 2–1246 of the State Government Article.

SECTION 3. AND BE IT FURTHER ENACTED, That Section 1 of this Act shall take effect October 1, 2019.

SECTION 4. AND BE IT FURTHER ENACTED, That, except as provided in Section 3 of this Act, this Act shall take effect July 1, 2019. Section 2 of this Act shall remain effective for a period of 1 year and, at the end of June 30, 2020, Section 2 of this Act, with no further action required by the General Assembly, shall be abrogated and of no further force and effect. Enacted under Article II, § 17(c) of the Maryland Constitution, May 25, 2019.

more individuals and organizations involved builds collective power on behalf of the issue and can illustrate broad and visible support.

Partnership with my state senator was crucial to build support both within the legislature and in the child advocacy ecosystem. Although he sought cosponsors including Delegate Brooke E. Lierman on the House side and introduced the legislation at the state house a few weeks later (House Bill 520/Senate Bill 406, **Box 3**), I shared the bill and sought partnership with other child advocacy organizations including the Maryland Chapter of the American Academy of Pediatrics (AAP), as well the state section of the American College of Obstetricians and Gynecologists (ACOG). In February 2019, the Congressional committee held a public hearing. I wrote testimony in support of the bill and recruited other organizations, including the Maryland AAP, to also submit testimony. I traveled to Annapolis to testify and met with supporters of the legislation. Several organizations that wished to be included in the proposed task force offered amendments, further building support.

The legislation passed both the House of Delegates and the Maryland Senate, and Governor Hogan signed it into law. The Task Force on Maryland Maternal and Child Health (Task Force) was established by Chapters 661 and 662 of the Acts of 2019 (House Bill 520/Senate Bill 406). A few weeks later, a Maryland Department of Health leader called to ask for advice on formation of the Maryland Maternal Child Health Task Force. The Chair of Pediatrics at the University of Maryland and I, as Chair of Pediatrics at Johns Hopkins University, were seated as Chair and Vice Chair of the task force. Task Force members included representatives from several state agencies, including the Maryland Department of Health, Maryland Department of Human Services, Maryland Medical Assistance Program, and HSCRC. The task force also included several other professional organizations: the Maryland Affiliate of the American College of Nurse Midwives, Maryland Association for the Treatment of Opioid Dependence, Maryland Chapter of the American Academy of Pediatrics, Maryland Patient Safety Center, and Maryland Section of the American College of Obstetricians and Gynecologists. To ensure broader responsiveness and accountability, the task force also included a community pediatrician, a representative from a community organization serving mothers and children, and 3 participants in targeted programs within the current care coordination system.

The task force met 10 times during 8 months and had a series of expert speakers and public discussions on recommendations to strengthen MCH. The work coordinated with other concurrent efforts including the Senate President's Workgroup on Equity and Inclusion, as well as Maryland's Maternal Mortality Review Committee

---

Box 4
Maryland Maternal and Child Health Task Force Recommendations.

Recommendation #1

Make MCH the third goal under the population health domain of Maryland's Integrated Health Improvement Strategy with the Centers for Medicare and Medicaid Services (CMS), with a focus on reducing maternal and infant mortality and fostering child and family mental, emotional, and behavioral health. Ensure that the strategy's first two goals under the population health domain, diabetes, and opioid/substance use disorder, include the MCH population.

Recommendation #2

Establish a standing Maternal and Child Health Committee (Committee) in the Maryland Department of Health (MDH) to develop a Blueprint for MCH and shared accountability framework that provides a roadmap to achieving outcome goals. This committee would develop an action plan, implement strategies, and define and monitor outcomes to improve MCH and eliminate racial/ethnic and socioeconomic disparities.

Recommendation #3

Ensure that the Maternal and Child Health Committee define, collect, and track process and outcome metrics throughout the care delivery system for the MCH population, to improve data utilization, data quality, and population health management, and to monitor progress toward high-priority outcomes relevant to MCH.

Recommendation #4

Tailor financing and payment models to the MCH population including establishment of a Maternal and Child Health Payment Advisory Subcommittee of the Maternal and Child Health Committee (see Recommendation #2). It should advise MDH and HSCRC on care delivery models and payment methodologies across the care delivery system that ensure quality and outcomes for the MCH population. This includes focus on Medicaid and commercial insurer policies, care transformation initiatives across the delivery system, incentivizing hospitals to invest in MCH care and population health programs, and creating MCH regional partnerships.

Recommendation #5

Extend Medicaid coverage for pregnant women until 12 months postpartum and provide care coordination and health literacy education for individuals as they transition coverage.

Recommendation #6

Ensure all pregnant women receive comprehensive prenatal care (PNC) by increasing awareness of and access to resources for all women, including a statewide Emergency Medicaid Program that covers undocumented immigrants.

Recommendation #7

Strengthen the obstetric workforce by further integrating Certified Nurse Midwives (CNMs) into Maryland Hospitals.

Recommendation #8

Foster healthy mental, emotional, and behavioral development of children and coordinate care to address MCH population health needs.

Recommendation #9

Ensure that Statewide MCH strategies and programs prioritize parent and community engagement, two-generation family approaches, and place-based outreach initiatives. Important components of these efforts are explicitly supporting families in their psychosocial needs and reaching children and families in community locations, including childcare centers and schools.

---

and others. Partnering with these constituencies was very important for coalition-building on the task force report and future legislation. Recommendations from their reports and activities were considered by the task force.

The final report was sent in August 2020 to the Maryland Speaker of the House and Maryland Senate President Bill Ferguson. Bill Ferguson, the state senator who had invited me to write the legislation months earlier and originally introduced the bill, had ascended to the Senate Presidency. Recommendations from the report are seen in **Box 4**.

STEP 4: COMMUNICATE THE MESSAGE

Dissemination of the message takes purposeful effort and involves multiple modalities and target audiences. Media advocacy may involve newspapers, magazines, websites, social media, television, and radio. Communications may be print-based (newsletters, op-eds, flyers, policy briefs), Internet-based (websites, email lists, blogs, social media), or in person (public speaking, professional meetings, meetings with legislators).

Although writing the report was a heavy lift, the work to disseminate and implement the recommendations was just starting. With support from the original bill sponsors, a press conference and congressional briefing were held in September 2020. With the bill's cosponsor from the Maryland House of Delegates, Brooke E. Lierman, we published an op-ed in the state's leading newspaper, the *Baltimore Sun*, entitled "Healthy Lives Begin Before Birth" in April 2021.[9] Local news outlets were frequently very receptive to communications from pediatric clinicians, academic institutions, and local legislators. Submitting online was easy and turnaround was fast, in contrast to academic publications.

Building on this foundation of publicity for the legislation and task force recommendations, the next steps were to disseminate the ideas widely and start on implementation. To do this, we pursued 2 areas of work: (1) advocacy to include MCH as the third population health priority in the Statewide Integrated Health Improvement Strategy (SIHIS) and (2) additional legislation to implement task force recommendations.

The first task force recommendation was for Maryland to name MCH as its third population health priority in its SIHIS, which guides state programming and funding. This was a key challenge and high hurdle. The Total Cost of Care Model in Maryland involved collaboration between the state and the Centers for Medicare and Medicaid Services' Innovation Center (CMMI) to specify the domains of health-care quality and delivery that the state would affect. A 2019 memorandum between the state and CMMI required Maryland to submit their SIHIS proposal to CMMI by December 31, 2020 outlining goals, measures, milestones, and targets proposed by the state to advance hospital quality, health-care transformation, and total population health.

Maryland Department of Health had already begun work and invested in 2 statewide population health priorities: diabetes and opioids. They were considering the third priority at the time the task force report came out. Despite task force recommendations, it was not at all a given that the third population priority would be MCH. Meetings were held with the Maryland Department of Health leadership and letters written. There was opposition from some hospitals and organizations who had little involvement with the MCH population, felt unprepared, or were concerned about the ability to improve MCH outcomes. Others wanted a different priority area. Having a thick skin to criticism, tenacity, and tough-minded continuing advocacy were required. It included legislator encouragement to name MCH as the third priority area and to include MCH in the other 2 population health priorities. We collaborated with the Department of Health to define MCH goals and specific metrics. At the end of December 2020, the state submitted the SIHIS to CMMI including MCH as the third population health priority specifying goals in reducing severe maternal morbidity and childhood asthma (https://hscrc.maryland.gov/Documents/Modernization/SIHIS%20Proposal%20-%

20CMMI%20Submission%2012142020.pdf). Although we would have liked to focus on MCH beyond maternal morbidity and childhood asthma, it was a start. CMMI approved the state's submission in March 2021.

In July 2021, the Governor announced the launch of a US$72 million Maternal and Child Health Care Initiative focused on prevention, early intervention, and addressing health disparities https://governor.maryland.gov/2021/07/06/governor-hogan-announces-launch-of-72-million-maternal-and-child-health-care-initiative/. HSCRC designated funds for both new statewide programs and expansion of existing health-care services, many mentioned in the task force report. These services include pilot expansion of home visiting services, reimbursement for doula services, innovative models of care such as CenteringPregnancy and Healthy Steps, expansion of the maternal opioid misuse model, initiatives to improve asthma outcomes and disparities, and initiatives to address disparities in maternal health.

The second area of implementation advocacy involved additional legislation supporting task force recommendations in the next 2021 Maryland legislative session. Task force recommendation #5 was to extend Medicaid coverage for pregnant women until 12 months postpartum and provide care coordination and health literacy education for individuals as they transition coverage. The legislature passed Senate Bill 923, which extended Medicaid coverage for comprehensive medical, dental, and other health care services for mothers from 2 to 12 months postpartum and widened eligibility. The legislation provided an estimated US$17 million in additional funding to improve health for mothers who participate in Maryland's Medicaid program.

Task force recommendation #8 was to foster healthy mental, emotional, and behavioral development of children and coordinate care to address MCH population health needs. Amid the current child mental health crisis that began before the pandemic, this recommendation received attention in passing House Bill 548–Trauma-Informed Care–Commission and Training (Healing Maryland's Trauma Act). The legislation called for a commission to coordinate a statewide initiative to prioritize the trauma-responsive and trauma-informed delivery of State services that affect children, youth, families, and older adults. The commission, in consultation with specified entities, must study and implement an Adverse Childhood Experiences Aware program.

Additional legislation included passage of the Maryland Prenatal and Infant Care Grant Program Fund for care coordination; the Maryland Health Equity Resource Act designating "Health Equity Resource Communities" to target State resources to specific areas to reduce health disparities, improve health outcomes, promote prevention services, and reduce health care costs; the Finance Maryland Health Equity Resource Act providing grants to address health disparities; and expanded Medicaid oral health prevention services.

Despite many successes, the story never ends and communicating the message continues. Each step of the way required continued vigilance and tenacity by many advocates to disseminate and implement the recommendations and keep MCH issues on the radar on the state level and at health-care institutions.

Children are our greatest resource and are the message we send to the future. Making sure children are healthy, ready to learn and on a trajectory to healthy adulthood must be our highest priority.

LESSONS LEARNED

To identify lessons from this case, it is helpful to consider the framework of 7 "Leadership Lessons Learned" by Steve Schroeder, MD, a past president of the Robert Wood Johnson Foundation:[10]

1. *Mission matters:* Our mission is to ensure the health and well-being of children, adolescents, and families toward excellent and equitable outcomes. Advocating for those who cannot speak for themselves, those that represent our future, and those from marginalized populations are special responsibilities. Our mission is noble; it resonates powerfully and on a personal level. Invite your legislators to come visit your workplace and talk with children, adolescents, and families.
2. *Focus is critical:* Focusing on specific solutions is critical. Hone the message (eg, "children are our future") and the ask. Although there are so many areas in MCH that need attention, "choosing your battles" is necessary. The task force had too many original recommendations and had to focus on specific actions and a reasonable number of solutions.
3. *Execution trumps strategy:* The quest for change does not end with the publication of an article, the start of a program, or the passing of a bill. Execution of the strategy requires dissemination, implementation, relationships, buy-in, and enforcement. Although this case involved introducing legislation and a task force during a 21-month period, continued work to implement task force recommendations and additional legislation were essential for the efforts to ultimately reach children, youth, and families.
4. *Social change comes hard:* Fairness and equity require dogged advocacy. In Maryland, we wished to raise attention to the critical needs of mothers and children, especially among those in low income and minoritized communities, and to change policies that disempower these populations. Although elevating MCH seems like "motherhood and apple pie," there was opposition to choosing MCH as a priority. Thick skin and tenacity are necessary. As clinicians, we know that improving health requires addressing political, environmental, and social determinants.
5. *Know when to hold them, know when to fold them:* If you do not succeed, try again. Timing and context are important. In this case, we had the opportunity to address the issue at a time and in a way that resonated. We were prepared to fold and try again if the bill did not pass the first time. Persistence is needed, and it pays off.
6. *Establish a strong internal culture:* Surround yourself with like-minded advocates. Build relationships and form coalitions. In Maryland, we found strong legislative partners who were passionate advocates. Advocacy is inherently a team sport.
7. *Pursue accountability:* In Maryland, we knew we needed to do more to address the needs of children, youth, and families and to ensure health equity. It was important to hold ourselves accountable to improve outcomes, which meant advocacy outside our offices. Hold yourself and others accountable to work toward change and making a difference. Our children and our future depend on it.

DISCLOSURE

No financial assistance was received to support this article. This study is original, not previously published, and not submitted for publication or consideration elsewhere.

Cheng: No disclosures of financial ties or potential/perceived conflicts of interest. She conceptualized and wrote the article, revised each draft, and approved the final article.

ACKNOWLEDGMENTS

■ Thanks to the team of maternal child advocates including legislative leaders that contributed to this work.

REFERENCES

1. Hahn H, Lou C, Isaacs JB, et al. Kids' share 2020: report on federal expenditures on children through 2019 and future projections. Urban Institute; 2020. Available at: https://www.urban.org/sites/default/files/publication/102614/kids-share-2020-chartbook_0.pdf. Accessed June 29, 2022.
2. Dieleman JL, Cao J, Chapin A, et al. US Health care spending by payer and health condition, 1996-2016. JAMA 2020;323(9):863–84.
3. National Academies of Sciences, Engineering, and Medicine. A roadmap to reducing child poverty. Washington, DC: The National Academies Press; 2019.
4. Garcia JL, Heckman JJ, Leaf DE, et al. NBER Working Paper No. 23479 June 2017, Revised February 2019 JEL No. C93,I28,J13, Available at: https://heckmanequation.org/www/assets/2017/01/w23479.pdf. Accessed June 26, 2022.
5. Heckman JJ. Invest in early childhood development: reduce deficits, strengthen the economy. 2013. Available at: https://heckmanequation.org/www/assets/2013/07/F_HeckmanDeficitPieceCUSTOM-Generic_052714-3-1.pdf. Accessed June 26, 2022.
6. Simmonds M, Llewellyn A, Owen CG, et al. Predicting adult obesity from childhood obesity: a systematic review and meta-analysis. Obes Rev 2016;17(2):95–107.
7. The National Center on Addiction and Substance Abuse at Columbia University, Adolescent Substance Use: America's #1 Public Health Problem. 2011. Available at: https://drugfree.org/reports/adolescent-substance-use-americas-1-public-health-problem/. Accessed June 26, 2022.
8. American Academy of Pediatrics. Advocacy Guide: pointing you in the right direction to become an effective advocate. American Academy of Pediatrics; 2009.
9. Lierman B, Cheng TL. Maternal Child Health forms the foundation for healthy and thriving lives. Baltimore Sun. 2021. 11. Available at: https://www.baltimoresun.com/opinion/op-ed/bs-ed-op-0426-maternal-child-health-20210426-wfq23bojsnfivcpuj3ywb7w4qq-story.html. Accessed June 26, 2022.
10. Schroeder S. Robert wood johnson foundation 2002 annual report. Available at: https://www.rwjf.org/en/library/annual-reports/annual-report-2002-.html. Accessed May 24, 22.
11. Bauer L. Brookings Institution. The COVID-19 crisis has already left too many children hungry in America. 2020. https://www.brookings.edu/blog/up-front/2020/05/06/the-covid-19-crisis-has-already-left-too-many-children-hungry-in-america/. [Accessed 22 October 2022].
12. Xie XY, Xue Q, Zhou Y, et al. Mental health status among children in home confinement during the coronavirus disease 2019 outbreak in Hubei Province, China. JAMA Pediatr 2020;174(9):898–900.
13. Parolin Z, Wimer C. Forecasting estimates of poverty during the COVID-19 crisis. Poverty & Social Policy Brief. 2020. 4(6):1-18. Available at: https://static1.squarespace.com/static/5743308460b5e922a25a6dc7/t/5e9786f17c4b4e20ca02d16b/1586988788821/Forecasting-Poverty-Estimates-COVID19-CPSP-2020.pdf.
14. Kids Count Data Center. Children in Poverty by Race/Ethnicity. 2018 data. Available at: https://datacenter.kidscount.org/. Accessed February 9, 2020.
15. Semega J, Kollar M, Creamer J, et al. U.S. Census bureau, current population reports, p60-266, income and poverty in the United States: 2018. Washington, DC:

U.S. Government Printing Office; 2019. Available at: https://www.census.gov/content/dam/Census/library/publications/2019/demo/p60-266.pdf.

16. Lesley B. Voices4Kids. The COVID-19 crisis is catastrophic for children too. 2020. Available at: https://medium.com/voices4kids/the-covid-19-crisis-is-catastrophic-for-children-too-572953c1eef9. Accessed April 15, 2020.

17. UNICEF Office of Research. Children of the Recession: the impact of the economic crisis on child well-being in rich countries, Innocenti Report Card 12. Florence: UNICEF Office of Research; 2014.

18. America's Health Rankings analysis of CDC WONDER online database, mortality files 2017, united health foundation. Available at: AmericasHealthRankings.org. Accessed February 9, 2020.

19. Maryland Department of Health. Maryland maternal mortality review 2019 annual report. Available at: https://phpa.health.maryland.gov/mch/Documents/Health-General%20Article,%20%C2%A713-1207,%20Annotated%20Code%20of%20Maryland%20-%202019%20Annual%20Report%20%E2%80%93%20Maryland%20Maternal%20Mortality%20Review.pdf. Accessed May 19, 2020.

20. America's Health Rankings analysis of CDC WONDER Online Database. Linked Birth/Infant Death files, United Health Foundation. Available at: AmericasHealthRankings.org. Accessed February 9, 2020.

21. Lo CB, Bridge JA, Shi J, et al. Children's mental health emergency department visits: 2007–2016. Pediatrics 2020;145(6):e20191536.

22. National Academies of Sciences. Engineering, and Medicine. In: Fostering Healthy Mental, Emotional, and Behavioral Development in Children and Youth: A National Agenda. Washington, DC: The National Academies Press; 2019.

23. Luca DL, Margiotta C, Staatz C, et al. Financial toll of untreated perinatal mood and anxiety disorders among 2017 births in the United States. Am J Public Health 2020;110(6):888–96.

24. Office of Disease Prevention and Health Promotion. Healthy People. 2020. Available at: https://www.healthypeople.gov/2020/topics-objectives/topic/maternal-infant-and-child-health. Accessed April 10, 2020.

25. Braveman P, Barclay C. Health disparities beginning in childhood: a life-course perspective. Pediatrics 2009;124(Suppl 3):S163–75.

26. Halfon N, Forrest CB, Lerner RM, et al. Handbook of life course health development. Cham: Springer; 2018.

27. Gluckman PD, Hanson MA, Cooper C, et al. Effect of in utero and early-life conditions on adult health and disease. N Engl J Med 2008;359(1):61–73.

28. Finkelstein EA, Graham WCK, Malhotra R. Lifetime direct medical costs of childhood obesity. Pediatrics 2014;133(5):854–62.

Firearm Injury Prevention Advocacy
Lessons Learned and Future Directions

Deanna Behrens, MSME, MD[a],*, Maya Haasz, MD[b],
James Dodington, MD[c], Lois K. Lee, MD, MPH[d]

KEYWORDS

- Firearm • Injury prevention • Legislative advocacy • Harm reduction

KEY POINTS

- A multi-pronged public health approach is needed to reduce the burden of injuries and deaths due to firearms.
- Pediatric clinicians are powerful advocates to advance legislation and policies to reduce harm due to firearms.
- To be effective advocates, it is important to form relationships with elected officials and key stakeholders.

INTRODUCTION

There are many paths for pediatric clinicians to be effective advocates. This article uses firearm injury prevention to present several examples of clinician advocacy. Firearms are the leading cause of injury death in children and youth 1 to 24 year old, overtaking motor vehicle traffic deaths in 2017 (**Fig. 1**).[1] Approximately two-thirds of firearm deaths are homicides, one-third are suicide, and a small proportion are due to unintentional shootings. For nonfatal firearm injuries approximately 80% are due to intentional assaults and 20% are due to unintentional shootings (**Fig. 2**).[1] Systemic racism and poverty have led to disparities in firearm injuries and death by sex, race, ethnicity, and socioeconomic environment.[2,3]

Data from a 2021 nationally representative survey reported 40% of US households with children had at least one firearm. This equates to an estimated 30 million children living in households with firearms. Among these households, 15% reported storing

[a] Division of Pediatric Critical Care, Department of Pediatrics, Advocate Children's Hospital, 1675 Dempster Street, Park Ridge, IL 60068, USA; [b] Section of Emergency Medicine, Children's Hospital Colorado, 13123 East 16th Avenue, Box 251, Aurora, CO 80045, USA; [c] Section of Pediatric Emergency Medicine, Yale School of Medicine, 100 York Street, Suite 1F, New Haven, CT 06511, USA; [d] Division of Emergency Medicine, Boston Children's Hospital, 300 Longwood Avenue, Boston, MA 02115, USA
* Corresponding author.
E-mail address: deanna.behrens@aah.org

Pediatr Clin N Am 70 (2023) 67–82
https://doi.org/10.1016/j.pcl.2022.09.002
0031-3955/23/© 2022 Elsevier Inc. All rights reserved.

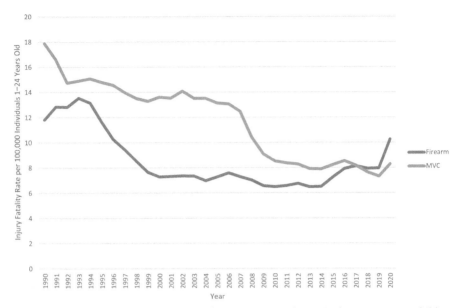

Fig. 1. Motor vehicle traffic and firearm fatality rates in the United States among children and youth 1–24 years old from 1990 to 2020. (*Data from* the Centers for Disease Control and Prevention, WISQARS (Web-Based Injury Statistics Query and Reporting System) (https://www.cdc.gov/injury/wisqars/index.html). Figure created by Katherine Douglas, MD.[1])

firearms loaded and unlocked, the least safe way to store firearms, for an estimated 4.6 million children living with firearms stored in this manner.[4]

A public health approach similar to that used to enhance motor vehicle safety must be applied to reverse the current upward trend of firearm injuries and deaths to US children and youth.[5] Legislation is one essential part of a multi-pronged approach for firearm harm reduction (**Table 1**). State-based firearm legislation varies widely across the United States (**Fig. 3**),[6] with more restrictive firearm laws associated with decreased state-level firearm death rates.[7] Clinician advocacy for effective legislation and policies to decrease firearm injuries and deaths in children and youth is critical to address this public health epidemic.[8] In this article we will describe three case studies of advocacy focused on firearm injury prevention at the individual, state, and federal levels.

Case Study: An Individual's Development as an Advocate for Firearm Harm Prevention Policies

As a pediatric intensivist at a large community hospital, I have directly witnessed the devastating effects of firearm violence. These patients require high critical care resource utilization with prolonged mechanical ventilation, surgical procedures, and blood product use leading to substantial healthcare costs in both the acute and chronic phases.[9] The mortality rate in patients admitted to the pediatric intensive care unit (PICU) due to firearm injuries is five times higher than the average PICU patient, and only 10% of survivors have good overall outcomes on discharge.[10]

Owing to my clinical experiences, the focus of my advocacy work is firearm injury prevention.

By attending the American Academy of Pediatrics (AAP) Advocacy Conference, working with my hospital's government relations team, and becoming an active

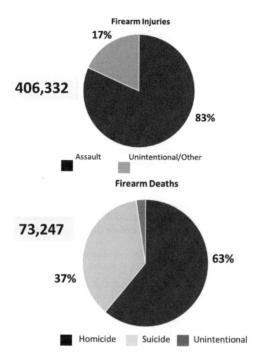

Fig. 2. Firearm injuries and deaths by intent and children and youth 1–24 years old in the United States from 2011 to 2020 (*N* = 479,579.). (*Data from* the Centers for Disease Control and Prevention, WISQARS (Web-Based Injury Statistics Query and Reporting System) (https://www.cdc.gov/injury/wisqars/index.html).[1])

participant in the Illinois Chapter of the American Academy of Pediatrics (ICAAP), I had been successful in my advocacy efforts. To affect change on a larger scale, I recognized the value of pursuing formal training in advocacy skills. I applied for and was accepted into the Academic Pediatric Association's (APA) Health Policy Scholars Program (HPSP). This is a 3-year longitudinal faculty development program focused on training pediatric clinicians to have successful careers in academic advocacy and policy with the goal of influencing policy at all levels.

Firearm injuries are the leading cause of death for children ages 1 to 17 year old in Illinois.[11] The Illinois Child Access Prevention (CAP) law states it is a Class C misdemeanor if a child younger than 14 year old accesses and uses a firearm to cause death or great bodily harm.[12] My initial project for the HPSP was to advocate for a stronger Illinois CAP law.

At the beginning of my firearm injury prevention advocacy efforts, I met with both my local mentor and national advisor to discuss how to reduce the burden of firearm injury on Illinois children. We worked with a team of stakeholders, including physicians and representatives from children's hospitals throughout the state, ICAAP, Strengthening Chicago's Youth (SCY), the Illinois Department of Public Health, and the Illinois State Medical Society. Through this coalition, we connected with a group of seven elected officials from the Illinois General Assembly who comprised the Gun Violence Prevention (GVP) caucus and convened a working group to advance legislation on this issue.

We encountered substantial barriers early in the process. The upcoming legislative cycle directly preceded an election year and was the first after redistricting following

Table 1	
State laws that could reduce firearm violence in the United States	
Specific Law	**Description of the Law**
Assault Weapons Bans	This law would restrict access to firearms, which are capable of injuring or killing the most people at one time, without the shooter having to reload the firearm.
Buyer Safety Regulations	This would require firearm buyers to obtain a permit or license to purchase a firearm, would require background checks, and/or mandate safety training. These laws could also address age limits for the purchase of certain types of long guns (eg, semi-automatic military style weapons).
CAP Laws	These laws regulate the safer storage of firearms by holding firearm owners liable if a child accesses (less restrictive) or could potentially access (more restrictive) a firearm. Negligence type CAP laws prohibit a firearm owner from intentionally, knowingly, or recklessly allowing a minor to access a firearm. The weakest of this type of law permits liability only if the firearm owner provides the firearm to a minor knowing there is a substantial risk the minor will use it.
ERPO Laws	These laws remove access (either possession and/or purchase) of firearms for an individual at risk for harming themselves or someone else. These orders are issued by a judge for a finite period of time (can last up to 1 year). Depending on the state, law enforcement, household members, friends, mental health professionals, coworkers, educators or school administrators can petition for an ERPO.
Limiting Numbers of Firearms Purchased within a Specific Time Period	This type of law might reduce illegal gun trafficking and the ability to build arsenals in a short period of time, for example, by limiting purchases to one firearm per month for an individual.
Universal Background Checks	These laws could require a more in-depth background check, including with information from local law enforcement as well as federal sources, for all individuals who lawfully take possession of a firearm. This would include not only sales from federally licensed dealers, but also at gun shows and between individuals. Ideally transaction records should be kept.

Data from Azad HA, Monuteaux MC, Rees CA, et al. Child Access Prevention Firearm Laws and Firearm Fatalities among Children Aged 0 to 14 Years, 1991-2016. *JAMA Pediatrics.* 2020;174(5):463-469. https://doi.org/10.1001/jamapediatrics.2019.6227; Madeira J. Firearm Legislation and Advocacy. In: *Pediatric Firearm Injuries and Fatalities: The Clinician's Guide to Policies and Approaches to Firearm Harm Prevention*; 2021:193-211; Santaella-Tenorio J, Cerda M, Vellaveces A, Galea S. What Do We Know About the Association Between Firearm Legislation and Firearm-Related Injuries? *Epidemiol Rev.* 2016;38:140-157.

the 2020 Census. In addition, the working days for the 2022 General Assembly were reduced due to the COVID-19 pandemic. Owing to these factors, the legislators felt it was extremely unlikely to pass any controversial GVP bills during this session. Despite this, the group remained optimistic about drafting and passing different legislation. We spent the next several months researching successful public health campaigns and messaging tools to provide an evidence-based approach to craft a statewide safer storage campaign. This focused on including sustained communication over time, messages paired with information about enforcements and incentives, and geographic and cultural considerations. The bill, HB4729 DPH Safe Gun Storage Campaign, included funding for firearm buy-back programs, a pilot study for firearm

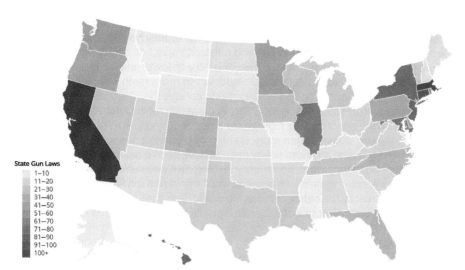

Fig. 3. Number of firearm laws by state in the United States in 2022. (The Changing Landscape of U.S. Gun Policy, STATE FIREARM LAWS 1991–2016, http://statefirearmlaws.org/.)

lock distribution, educational materials for pediatric providers, and funding for an evaluative component.

Although the bill had bipartisan support, it was still important to recruit additional allies. We created a one-pager about the bill, contacted the government relations teams at every children's hospital in the state, and sent out advocacy action alerts. We presented the bill to the Children's Health Caucus, a bipartisan group of Illinois Senators and Representatives. I developed a relationship with my state representative, and she cosponsored this bill along with 28 other state representatives. Over 30 supporting organizations signed the bill, including every major children's hospital in the state, state and local public health departments, and community groups. On June 10, 2022, Governor Pritzker signed the bill into Illinois state law.[13]

Parallel to the work in the GVP group and the safer storage campaign, we have been working to develop an advocacy curriculum for fellows with the AAP's Section on Critical Care. I also published an invited editorial about firearm violence in the *Pediatric Critical Care Medicine* (*PCCM*) journal in response to the first article ever published in *PCCM* about firearms. In the corresponding editorial, we wrote: "When we searched the archives of *PCCM* for past publications on firearm violence, the "best matches" for firearm and gun were forearm and gut, but this is changing."[14]

Case Study: State-Level Advocacy—The Colorado Experience

On April 20, 1999, two high-school seniors at Columbine High School in Littleton, Colorado arrived at their school armed with shotguns, a semi-automatic handgun, and a variety of bombs. The pair embarked on a shooting rampage, killing 13 and injuring 24, before killing themselves. The Columbine shooting was the deadliest high school shooting the United States had every experienced up until that time and remains the deadliest mass shooting in Colorado.[15] This tragedy sparked discussions surrounding firearm laws locally and nationally.

In Colorado, the firearm fatality rate for children and youth (1–24 year old) in 2020 was 10.6 per 100,000, similar to the national average. Fifty eight percent of deaths were due to suicide, 36% homicide, and the remaining deaths were unintentional or of undetermined intent.[16] Colorado also ranks fifth in the country for mass shooting deaths,[17] with 52 deaths and 125 injuries in nine mass shootings since 1993.[15] Although mass shootings account for less than 1% of Colorado's firearm deaths, they can have broader impact due to their large-scale media attention and outsized impact on communities.

More restrictive state firearm laws are associated with lower rates of firearm injury and deaths in children and young adults. Colorado, which ranks tenth in the country for the strength of its firearm laws,[18] has taken decades to achieve this. Changes to firearm legislation were frequently catalyzed by local events garnering media attention (**Fig. 4**). Many of these laws were enacted after high profile mass shootings, which can draw greater attention to firearm violence than more commonly occurring homicides and suicides. Successes in advancing a firearm safety agenda have been a result of changes in legislative makeup, advocacy work, community involvement and current events. Moreover, Colorado has several organizations focused wholly, or in part, on firearm legislation, education, and outreach. The oldest of these, Colorado Ceasefire, has been pivotal in advocating for, and bringing about, safer firearm legislation since its inception 2000.[19]

After Columbine, where the shooters obtained shotguns from a gun show, a bill to close the Gun Show Loophole (permitting sales at a gun show to proceed without a background check) was presented to the colorado general assembly (CGA). This bill failed narrowly, despite having broad popular support. A grassroots organization then obtained double the required signatures to put the question to a referendum via a citizen's initiative, which passed by a margin of 70% to 30% in 2000.[20] This was a stunning example of the power of advocacy among motivated citizens.

In Colorado pro-gun rights legislators held most seats in both the House and Senate until 2004. During this time firearm restrictions were loosened, with one law barring cities from enacting more restrictive firearm laws than the state (preemption), and another allowing for more permissive concealed carry.[21] Changing this landscape took time. A big change occurred in 2013 after the Aurora Theater Shooting, the largest US mass shooting (82 killed or injured)18 up until that time. That year, five new firearm laws were enacted including regulations expanding background checks and requiring in-person training for concealed carry. Notably, two state senators were recalled over their support of the laws and a third resigned to avoid recall.[22]

Within the next 8 years, many bills that would have loosened restrictions were defeated, and seven more laws passed, including Extreme Risk Protection Order (ERPO) and Safe Storage Laws. Physicians were staunch supporters of these laws, and made their voices heard at the CGA (Colorado General Assembly). In 2021, our pediatrician-initiated, hospital-based, Firearm Injury Prevention Group (FIPG) partnered with Colorado Ceasefire in supporting the Safe Storage and ERPO bills, writing letters to the editor and testifying at the CGA. Our clinical expertise complemented their legislative experience and knowledge, and this partnership was able to advance a very compelling case at the state level. Further, we collaborated with our hospital legislative team and Colorado AAP chapter, lending our position even more credibility and assuring legislators they had public support. Our efforts were designed to show strong support from pediatricians in advancing firearm legislation to legislators.

Case Study: State to Federal Level Advocacy for Ethan's Law

Pediatricians play a critical role in protecting our children. They are the first-line of defense.

That is why it is essential for pediatricians to be leading the way in promoting safe gun storage.

—Kristin Miller Song, Esq.

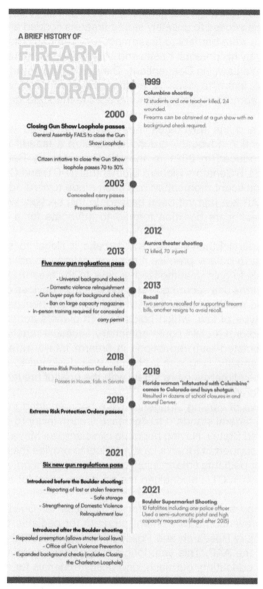

Fig. 4. History of firearms in Colorado. (Figure created using data from Colorado Ceasefire (https://www.coloradoceasefire.org).[18])

Case Background: Excerpt from Official Press Release of the State of Connecticut[23]

"Ethan Song, 15, of Guilford, CT, was shot and killed on January 31, 2018 while handling a .357 Magnum pistol at a neighbor's house. The pistol was one of three unattended firearms he and a friend knew were kept in a bedroom closet owned by the friend's father. The firearms were stored in a cardboard box inside of a large Tupperware container. While each of the weapons were secured with operable gun locks, the keys and ammunition for the firearms were located inside of the same box."

Stories are powerful. We know unintentional shootings and suicides occurring when children or youth gain access to unsafely stored firearms (loaded and unlocked) could be prevented if there were barriers to firearm access. The tragic death of Ethan Song catalyzed advocacy by his parents, Kristin and Mike Song, to create and pass a stronger CAP law, "Ethan's Law," in Connecticut. They brought a bipartisan group of lawmakers together to examine gaps in existing legislation and were able to gain significant support from community members across the state to pass Ethan's Law in 2019.[24]

Ethan's parents and the advocates they galvanized joined with other national firearm injury prevention advocacy groups to develop a federal version of Ethan's Law. This was introduced in 2021 to the US Congress by Representative Rosa DeLauro (D-CT) and US Senators Richard Blumenthal (D-CT) and Christopher Murphy (D-CT). Although significant momentum has been made toward advancing this legislation, no federal CAP law has yet been passed. In this section, we will examine the ways in which a healthcare coalition formed to advocate for a federal version of Ethan's Law.

The proposed federal Ethan's Law would make it illegal to store or keep any unsafely stored firearm on any premise if a minor, defined as an individual less than 18 years old, is likely to gain unauthorized access to the firearm. Further, it requires individuals with firearms use secure gun storage or safety devices or keep the firearm on their person. The most stringent type of CAP laws are negligence laws such as Ethan's Law. This type of law, which holds firearm owners accountable if firearms are not safely stored and a child could potentially access it regardless of the use of the firearm, is associated with reductions in firearm fatality rates in children 0 to 14 years old.[7] The specific language in the law was designed to encourage firearm owners to secure their firearms more safely with the goal of preventing these devastating events in children and youth.

Although CAP laws of varying stringency have been enacted in many states, it is important to have a federal standard to decrease firearm injury to children and youth throughout the United States. Having pediatric clinicians like Maya Haasz, MD, testify to the US Senate in support of Ethan's Law is critical to provide the pediatric expertise to garner support for pediatric firearm injury prevention legislation. As an advocate for child injury prevention in CT, I also joined the advocacy effort for a federal version of Ethan's Law.

In 2021 I joined as a Faculty Facilitator of Trainees for Child Injury Prevention (T4CIP), an injury prevention development program for pediatric trainees organized by the Center for Injury Research and Policy at Nationwide Children's Hospital with the sponsorship of the AAP. This year-long training program focuses on preparing trainees to develop education, outreach, and policy materials for national injury prevention advocacy campaigns (https://www.nationwidechildrens.org/research/areas-of-research/center-for-injury-research-and-policy/education-and-training/t4cip).[25]

The advocacy focus of T4CIP in fall 2021 was firearm injury prevention, including for a federal Ethan's Law. My T4CIP role was to assist in guiding the trainees in developing legislative and policy advocacy materials and to help organize the T4CIP Day of Action for firearm safety. We created two reference guides, which can be used locally and nationally. The first guide (**Fig. 5**) provides basic firearm injury statistics to paint the scope of the problem for legislators. It also includes policy opportunities to improve safer storage of firearms and funding for firearm injury education and research, as well as links to more in-depth resources. This provides a foundation for discussions about strengthening CAP laws with legislators. The second guide (**Figs. 6** and **7**) uses Ethan's Law as an example to provide a sample elevator pitch, which clinicians

How to Strengthen Local Firearm Safety Laws

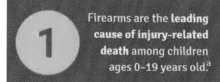

1 Firearms are the **leading cause of injury-related death** among children ages 0–19 years old.[a]

4X Black children and teens are **4 times more likely** than their White peers to die by firearms.[a]

A child or teen dies from a firearm every **2 hours and 34 minutes.**[a]

93% of parents would be comfortable with being asked about a firearm in their home.[b]

1. WISQARS Data Visualization. Accessed July 24, 2021. https://wisqars-viz.cdc.gov:8006/explore-data/home
2. ASK to End Family Fire. Brady. Accessed September 22, 2021. https://www.bradyunited.org/program/end-family-fire/asking-saves-kids

Priority Evidence-Based Policy Opportunities

	Child Access Prevention (CAP) & Incentivizing Safer Storage	Firearm Safety Screening & Education
Description	• Require safe storage measures to restrict access to guns by children • Address penalties for negligently storing a firearm unlocked and accessible to a child	• Promote pediatrician screening for firearms in the home • Make gun locks and other firearm safety tools and information more accessible
Importance & Related Research	• People who safely store their firearms are less likely to die by firearm suicide • States with CAP laws may help increase compliance with safe storage behaviors and have been shown to have reduced rates of gun suicides	• Screening and education related to firearm safety for children is an important injury prevention strategy similar to promoting child product safety (e.g. car seats, bike helmets) and safety on playgrounds and in pools
Recommended Action	• Each state needs to implement a Child Access Prevention law which incentivizes gun owners to securely store firearms locked and unloaded regardless of whether a child accesses and uses a gun • Contact your state representative and ask them to support passage of stronger child access prevention laws	• Increase public awareness of firearm safety effectiveness • Improve policies to address the disproportionate impact of gun violence on children and youth of color • Contact your state representative and ask them to support passage

Additional Resources

Fig. 5. How to strengthen local firearm safety laws. (With permission from T4CIP.)

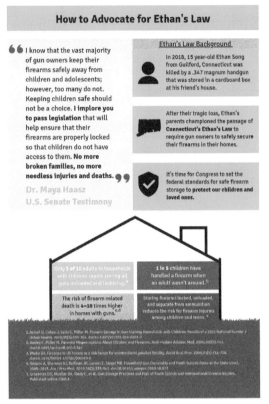

Fig. 6. How to advocate for firearm safety laws. (With permission from T4CIP.)

can use with legislators and their staff. It also includes links for finding local, state, and federal legislators. Our work culminated on October 26, 2021 with the T4CIP Day of Action, which was a virtual event involving hundreds of pediatric clinicians and over three million social media impressions.

Lessons Learned

Use available resources

Clinicians are powerful allies in legislative advocacy but may lack the formal training or confidence to pursue it. Available resources can be highly effective in supporting legislative advocacy. The AAP's annual Advocacy Conference is an effective introduction to legislative advocacy for the clinician, and often focuses on firearm injury prevention. These efforts, along with work of other AAP groups, have contributed to federal funding for firearm research for the first time in nearly a quarter of a century. For a deeper understanding of advocacy and research, pediatric clinicians can also pursue further education (eg, Masters of Public Health) or apply for the HPSP. Programs like T4CIP can support clinicians in building the skills needed in legislative advocacy and policy work.

Develop relationships and build partnerships

Rarely is legislative advocacy accomplished by one individual. Developing relationships with other clinicians, legislative officials, and various stakeholders is critical. There are many ways to form these networks, including social media, collaborating with hospital government relations team, engaging like-minded community

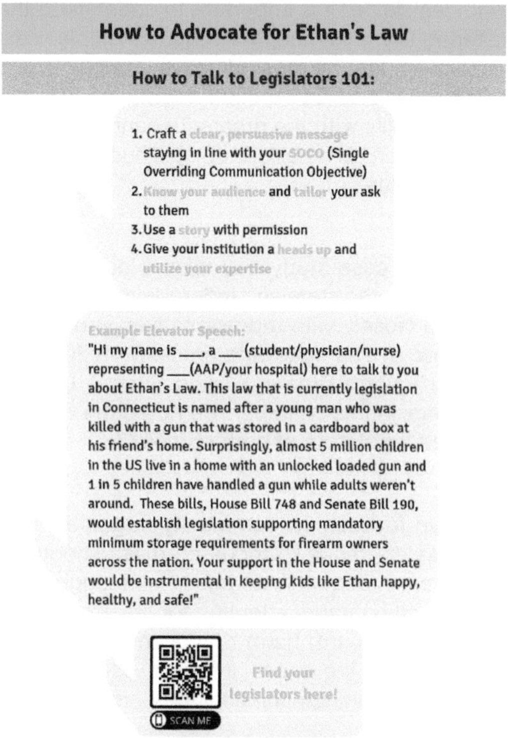

How to Advocate for Ethan's Law

How to Talk to Legislators 101:

1. Craft a clear, persuasive message staying in line with your SOCO (Single Overriding Communication Objective)
2. Know your audience and tailor your ask to them
3. Use a story with permission
4. Give your institution a heads up and utilize your expertise

Example Elevator Speech:

"Hi my name is ___, a ___ (student/physician/nurse) representing ___(AAP/your hospital) here to talk to you about Ethan's Law. This law that is currently legislation in Connecticut is named after a young man who was killed with a gun that was stored in a cardboard box at his friend's home. Surprisingly, almost 5 million children in the US live in a home with an unlocked loaded gun and 1 in 5 children have handled a gun while adults weren't around. These bills, House Bill 748 and Senate Bill 190, would establish legislation supporting mandatory minimum storage requirements for firearm owners across the nation. Your support in the House and Senate would be instrumental in keeping kids like Ethan happy, healthy, and safe!"

Find your legislators here!

Fig. 7. How to talk with legislators. (With permission from T4CIP.)

organizations, and working with state and national AAP chapters. By partnering with diverse stakeholders, clinicians can access other opportunities, including working directly with community leaders and those with lived experiences; producing work in other domains like Facebook Live or podcasts; and presenting to groups such as Moms Demand Action. Leveraging connections with the media to disseminate messaging is also important.

We recommend getting to know your legislative candidates and their views on firearm legislation, voting accordingly, and finding ways to support their campaigns. We also encourage clinicians to build relationships with your legislators, prepare one-page information sheets ("one-pagers") for them on proposed legislation, and be available to provide oral and/or written testimony. As pediatric clinicians, we are trusted experts and have powerful personal and patient stories to share. All of this assures legislators they have the support of their constituents, which has the potential to guide and facilitate their support for proposed firearm safety legislation.

Be flexible and patient while working with elected officials

Advocacy is an evolving process—it is often said that advocacy is a marathon, not a sprint. Persistence, the ability to move beyond rejection to keep trying, to be able to deflect negative reactions, and the willingness to be flexible and compromise are essential skills when conducting legislative advocacy, especially with an issue as political as firearms. Particularly in legislative advocacy, the political climate changes rapidly. We must be non-partisan and professional to work on advancing health policies affecting the health and well-being of children.

When partnering with legislators it is important to understand that multiple bills are unlikely to pass simultaneously, and many will require multiple sessions. It is essential to help prioritize which laws might be most effective and better received among constituents. In Illinois, Colorado, and Connecticut legislation was created by and with elected officials to advance bills with the greatest chance of success. Each success was an opportunity to work on other bills that continued to advance the legislative agenda of keeping children safe.

Bipartisan outreach matters

As in the Illinois and Colorado case-study examples, bipartisan support was essential for advancing this legislation at the state and federal level. For Ethan's Law in CT, Kristin and Mike Song worked closely with representatives in both parties to ensure the passage of the bill into law. In one statewide article from 2019, it was reported that Rep. Vincent Candelora (R-North Branford), said Ethan's Law was an example of the way we should do things in this chamber. He noted the bill came from dialogues, not confrontation, between legislators of both parties.[26]

Work with media

Although local media often focuses on community tragedies, national media attention surrounding firearm safety tends to focus on mass shootings, which represent only a small fraction of firearm deaths in all ages.[27] Although the aim is not to capitalize on tragedy, this publicity garners attention for firearm legislation and may facilitate further discussion about firearm harm reduction through legislation. Moreover, increased media attention on the more frequent causes of firearm injury and death—suicide, homicide, and unintentional injuries—may be important for proposing or supporting a bill.

Language is powerful

Recent work from public health leaders in firearm injury prevention makes it clear the language used in crafting communications regarding firearm safety is critical.[28] This is essential to ensure the message will be received and heard.[29] The language in Ethan's Law consistently uses the term "firearm" rather than "gun," which is important to influence harm reduction more broadly. In addition, the language focuses on how to keep children and teens safe in homes with firearms rather than decreasing or curtailing firearm ownership.

Prioritize equity

It is important that work is done through a lens to improve child health equity. Gun violence affects different group disproportionately, such as Black children,[30] particularly Black male adolescents, and children who live in poverty.[2] Victim-blaming and biased perception of effects of gun violence can lead to reduced sense of urgency to solve the underlying problems of systemic racism and poverty.[31]

Develop a thick skin

In the United States, conversations about firearm safety can become politically fraught. This can draw attention to advocates, particularly in avenues such as social media. The majority of the population supports measures to keep children safe. A recent poll by Morning Consult/Politico shows that 68% of voters support stricter gun control laws.[32] By remaining objective and professional and relying on existing evidence-based medicine, pediatricians can speak for the need of the patients and continue to advocate to reduce the burden of gun violence on children.

Future Directions for Advocacy

As deaths from firearms have increased among US children and youth to now become the number cause of death, a multi-pronged public health approach is necessary to reverse this trend. After the Dickey amendment was passed in 1996, the CDC and then other federal funding agencies, including the National Institutes of Health (NIH), were restricted from providing funding for firearm-related research. As a result, the science and researchers for firearm violence prevention now lag far behind other conditions.[8,9] In 2020, Congress appropriated funding for firearm research: $25 million divided between the NIH and CDC. Given the nearly quarter century without federal research funding, much more will be needed to rebuild research in this area. A sustained effort across multiple stakeholders will be essential to try to advance change. Some areas for future directions for advocacy include, but are not limited to:

- State and federal legislation: universal background check laws, comprehensive ERPO laws, increasing the age limit for purchase of specific types of firearms and ammunition
- Establishment of a federal agency tasked with firearm safety, like the National Highway Transportation Safety Administration (NHTSA) has the mission to make motor vehicles and roads safer to decrease motor vehicle injuries and deaths in the United States
- Increased research funding for firearm injury prevention
- Increased research and resources into eliminating underlying causes of disparities in firearm mortality in children who are Black or who live in poverty, such as systemic racism and concentrated areas of poverty.
- Patient/family level education and funding for safer firearm storage and lethal means counseling

SUMMARY

This article shows how pediatric clinicians are natural advocates with powerful stories who can partner with elected officials and grass-roots organizations to enact policy changes. In each case study, pediatricians developed coalitions with other stakeholders and built relationships with legislators and their staff to forward the agenda of decreasing firearm violence to children and youth. We are all stronger when working together, and the pediatric clinician voice in collaboration with other allies and stakeholders can be highly effective in promoting policies to advance child health, including for firearm injury prevention.

CLINICS CARE POINTS

- Gun violence is a public health crisis. In 2017, firearm injuries became the leading cause of death in children and adolescents 1-24 years old in the United States.
- To reduce the burden of firearm injuries and mortality on children, we need a multi-pronged strategy, similar to the approach used to decrease deaths due to motor vehicle crashes.
- Only the strongest Child Access Prevention Laws have been shown to decrease mortality.
- Children from marginalized racial and ethnic groups and those who live in poverty are disproportionately affected by gun violence.

ACKNOWLEDGMENTS

For creation of Figures: Katherine Douglas, MD. For contributions to Figures and T4CIP programming referenced in this publication: Gary Smith, MD, DRPH, Tracy Mehan, MA, Laura Dattner, MA, Scott Risney, and Hannah Hollon, MD. T4CIP is a program sponsored by the Center for Injury Research and Policy at The Abigail Wexner Research Institute at Nationwide Children's Hospital in Columbus, Ohio, and the American Academy of Pediatrics Section on Pediatric Trainees and Council on Injury, Violence, and Poison Prevention. The Centers for Disease Control and Prevention also provides funding for the Center for Injury Research and Policy at the Abigail Wexner Research Institute at Nationwide Chidlren's Hospital.

DISCLOSURE

Dr L.K. Lee receives royalties as an editor for the book, "Pediatric Firearm Injuries and Fatalities: The Clinician's Guide to Policies and Approaches to Firearm Harm Prevention."

REFERENCES

1. WISQARS (Web-based Injury Statistics Query and Reporting System)|Injury Center|CDC. Available at: https://www.cdc.gov/injury/wisqars/index.html. Accessed April 9, 2022.
2. Barrett JT, Lee LK, Monteaux MC, et al. Association of County-Level Poverty and Inequities with Firearm-Related Mortality in US Youth. JAMA Pediatr 2022;176(2). https://doi.org/10.1001/jamapediatrics.2021.4822.
3. Andrews AL, Killings X, Oddo ER, et al. Pediatric Firearm Injury Mortality Epidemiology. Pediatrics 2022;149(3). https://doi.org/10.1542/peds.2021-052739.
4. Miller M, Azrael D. Firearm Storage in US Households With Children. JAMA Netw Open 2022;5(2):e2148823.
5. Lee LK, Douglas K, Hemenway D. Crossing Lines — A Change in the Leading Cause of Death among U.S. Children. N Engl J Med 2022;386(16):1485–7. https://doi.org/10.1056/NEJMp2200169.
6. Siegel M. State-by-State Firearm Law Data | State Firearm Laws. State Firearm Laws. Available at: https://www.statefirearmlaws.org/. . Accessed April 9, 2022.
7. Azad HA, Monteaux MC, Rees CA, et al. Child Access Prevention Firearm Laws and Firearm Fatalities among Children Aged 0 to 14 Years, 1991-2016. JAMA Pediatr 2020;174(5):463–9. https://doi.org/10.1001/jamapediatrics.2019.6227.
8. Madeira J. Firearm legislation and advocacy. In: Lee L, Fleegler E, editors. Pediatric firearm injuries and fatalities: clinician's guide policies approaches firearm harm prev. Switzerland AG: Springer International Publishing; 2021. p. 193–211.
9. Kamat PP, Santore MT, Hoops KEM, et al. Critical care resource use, cost, and mortality associated with firearm-related injuries in US children's hospitals. J Pediatr Surg 2020;55(11):2475–9. https://doi.org/10.1016/j.jpedsurg.2020.02.016.
10. Bagdure D, Foster CB, Garber N, et al. Outcomes of Children With Firearm Injuries Admitted to the PICU in the United States. Pediatr Crit Care Med 2021;22(11):944–9. https://doi.org/10.1097/PCC.0000000000002785.
11. Everytown. Gun Violence in Illinois. Available at: https://everystat.org/wp-content/uploads/2021/02/Gun-Violence-in-Illinois-2.9.2021.pdf. Accessed February 23, 2022.

12. Illinois Legislative Reference Bureau. Illinois CAP Law (720 ILCS 5/24-9). https://www.ilga.gov/legislation/ilcs/fulltext.asp?DocName=072000050K24-9.   [Accessed 23 February 2022].

13. DPH - Safe Gun Storage. Illinois General Assembly; 2022.

14. Behrens DM, Hoops KEM. This Is Our Lane: The Role of Pediatric Intensivists in Firearm Violence and Injury Prevention. Pediatr Crit Care Med 2021;22(11). https://doi.org/10.1097/PCC.0000000000002797.

15. Hamm K. Tracking Colorado's mass shootings: 52 have died in nine incidents since 1993. The Denver Post. Available at: https://www.denverpost.com/2021/03/24/colorado-mass-shootings-incidents-list/. Accessed April 9, 2022.

16. WISQARS Data Visualization. CDC. Available at: https://wisqars.cdc.gov/data/non-fatal/home. Accessed March 19, 2022.

17. Mass shootings in the U.S. by state 1982-2022. Statista. Available at: https://www.statista.com/statistics/811541/mass-shootings-in-the-us-by-state/.   Accessed March 19, 2022.

18. Gun Safety Policies Save Lives | Everytown Research & Policy | Everytown Research & Policy. Everytown. Available at: https://everytownresearch.org/rankings/. Accessed March 19, 2022.

19. Ceasefire Colorado. Colorado Ceasefire. Available at: https://www.coloradoceasefire.org/. Accessed March 19, 2022.

20. Janofsky M. Colorado Panel Defeats Move to Close a Gun-Show Loophole - The New York Times. The New York Times. Available at: https://www.nytimes.com/2000/02/12/us/colorado-panel-defeats-move-to-close-a-gun-show-loophole.html. Accessed April 9, 2022.

21. Kopel D. Guns on university campuses: The Colorado experience - The Washington Post. The Washington Post. Available at: https://www.washingtonpost.com/news/volokh-conspiracy/wp/2015/04/20/guns-on-university-campuses-the-colorado-experience/. Accessed March 19, 2022.

22. Healy J. Colorado Lawmakers Ousted in Recall Vote Over Gun Law - The New York Times. The New York Times. Available at: https://www.nytimes.com/2013/09/11/us/colorado-lawmaker-concedes-defeat-in-recall-over-gun-law.html.   Accessed March 19, 2022.

23. Office of the Governor of Ned Lamont. Governor lamont signs Ethan's law to strengthen requirements on the safe storage of firearms in the home. Press Release from the Office of Governor Ned Lamont. Available at: https://portal.ct.gov/Office-of-the-Governor/News/Press-Releases/2019/06-2019/Governor-Lamont-Signs-Ethans-Law-to-Strengthen-Requirements-on-the-Safe-Storage-of-Firearms. Accessed April 9, 2022.

24. An Act Concerning the Safe Storage of Firearms in the Home and Firearm Safety Programs in Public Schools. Connecticut General Assembly; 2019.

25. Nationwide Children's Hospital. Trainees for Child Injury Prevention. T4CIP. Available at: https://www.nationwidechildrens.org/research/areas-of-research/center-for-injury-research-and-policy/education-and-training/t4cip. Accessed April 11, 2022.

26. Kramer J. CT gun safety law inspired by Guilford teen's death advances. Connecticut Post. Available at: https://www.ctpost.com/local/article/CT-gun-storage-law-inspired-by-Guilford-teen-s-13827287.php. Accessed April 9, 2022.

27. Rees CA, Lee LK, Fleegler EW, et al. Mass School Shootings in the United States: A Novel Root Cause Analysis Using Lay Press Reports. Clin Pediatr 2019;58(13):1423–8. https://doi.org/10.1177/0009922819873650.

28. Haasz M, Boggs JM, Beidas RS, et al. Firearms, physicians, families, and kids: finding words that work. J Pediatr 2022. https://doi.org/10.1016/j.jpeds.2022.05.029.

29. Betz ME, Harkavy-Friedman J, Loren Dreier F, et al. Talking About "Firearm Injury" and "Gun Violence": Words Matter. Am J Public Health 2021;111:2105–10.

30. Formica MK. An Eye on Disparities, Health Equity, and Racism—The Case of Firearm Injuries in Urban Youth in the United States and Globally. Pediatr Clin North Am 2021;68(2):389–99. https://doi.org/10.1016/j.pcl.2020.12.009.

31. Lee LK, Chaudhary S, Kemal S, et al. Addressing the void: firearm injury prevention in the USA. Lancet Child Adolesc Health. Published online May 2022. doi:10.1016/S2352-4642(22)00158-4

32. Voter Support for Stricter Gun Control Reaches New High - Morning Consult. https://morningconsult.com/2022/06/15/new-high-in-voter-support-for-stricter-gun-control-survey/. Accessed June 18, 2022.

Advocacy on the Federal Level

Inclusion of Children in Clinical Research

The Role of Advocacy and a Personal Journey

Scott C. Denne, MD[a],*, James Baumberger, MPP[b],
Lynn Olson, PhD[c]

KEYWORDS

• Clinical research • Inclusion • Advocacy • Children • Women

KEY POINTS

- Sustained advocacy over many years has been necessary to advance clinical research for children.
- Individuals can contribute to this advancement by embarking on a personal journey of advocacy.
- It is important to recognize that advocacy has long timelines and is rarely linear.
- Persistence, a focused ask, and working with experienced advocates can lead to success.

INTRODUCTION

Modern clinical research is less than 100 years old. In that time, there has been a constant effort at balancing human subjects' protections, minimizing risks, and providing access and inclusion to clinical trials. The importance and benefits of participating in clinical research have been increasingly recognized by the public, and vigorous advocacy efforts have been required to ensure full inclusion.

Unfortunately, there have been well-documented abuses in clinical research, including those of African Americans in the Tuskegee syphilis trial, and inappropriate studies of prisoners and institutionalized children.[1] In response to these abuses, there was a heightened focus on protecting human subjects participating in clinical research. This resulted in the Belmont report in 1974 that outlined the principles for the ethical conduct of clinical research.[2] A more robust system of institutional review

No disclosures.
[a] Indiana University School of Medicine, Riley Hospital for Children, 705 Riley Hospital Drive, RI 2606, Indianapolis, IN 46202, USA; [b] Federal Advocacy, American Academy of Pediatrics, 601 13th Street, NW Suite 400 North, Washington, DC 20005, USA; [c] American Academy of Pediatrics, 345 Park Boulevard, Itasca, IL 60143, USA
* Corresponding author.
E-mail address: sdenne@iu.edu

Pediatr Clin N Am 70 (2023) 83–90
https://doi.org/10.1016/j.pcl.2022.09.005
0031-3955/23/© 2022 Elsevier Inc. All rights reserved.

pediatric.theclinics.com

boards was implemented to better ensure these ethical principles were upheld.[1] However, efforts often went beyond the protection of human subjects in research and resulted in the protection of subjects *from* research.

WOMEN IN CLINICAL RESEARCH

Women in particular experienced being protected *from* research. In 1977, The US Food and Drug Administration (FDA) recommended that women of childbearing potential be excluded from early-phase clinical trials to protect a possible developing fetus.[3,4] This recommendation extended to women who were using birth control, who were single, or whose husbands were vasectomized. Although the FDA recommendation was for early-phase clinical trials, women were often excluded from all phases of clinical trials, including crucial human immunodeficiency virus studies and large cardiovascular trials.[5] These exclusions resulted in inadequate information about the efficacy and safety of many drugs used in women. Recognizing that clinical research has important benefits and risks, Women's Health advocacy groups began their efforts to better include women in clinical trials.[6] In 1986, the National Institutes of Health (NIH) established a policy to encourage investigators to include women in clinical trials. However, this policy resulted in little progress for inclusion, and advocacy groups pressed for congressional action.[6] The NIH Revitalization Act of 1993 (Public Law 103–43) required that the NIH ensure that "women and minorities" are included in clinical research.[7] The same year, the FDA explicitly reversed its recommendation excluding women of childbearing potential from early clinical trials.[4] In large part due to vigorous advocacy, the inclusion of women in clinical research has drastically improved.

HISTORY OF ADVOCACY FOR INCLUSION OF CHILDREN IN CLINICAL RESEARCH

Sustained advocacy has also been necessary to advance clinical research for children. For example, Robert Cook, MD, chair of Pediatrics at John Hopkins University in 1960 strongly urged the director of the NIH to make clinical research centers available to children.[8] However, his request was denied on the basis that results from adult studies could be used to extrapolate to children. Cook persevered, and with the support of multiple pediatric organizations, the NIH finally recognized the value of clinical trials in children. With presidential and congressional support, the National Institute of Child Health and Human Development (NICHD) was created in 1962.[9]

In October of 1962, President Kennedy said:

We will look to the National Institutes of Child Health and Human Development for a concentrated attack on the unsolved health problems of children and of the mother infant relationships. This legislation will encourage imaginative research into the complex processes of human development from conception to old age.

In 2007, by an act of Congress, NICHD renamed the *Eunice Kennedy Shriver* National Institute of Child Health and Human Development in honor of Mrs Shriver's long-term advocacy on behalf of people with intellectual and developmental disabilities.

In the years following the creation of NICHD, clinical trials in children funded by NIH focused primarily on specific diseases, in particular pediatric cancer. These trials had high participation rates that led to great success; childhood cancer was transformed from an essentially incurable disease to one with a combined 5-year survival rate of 80%.[10] Despite this remarkable success in pediatric cancer, continued advocacy by pediatricians and the public was required to ensure the wider inclusion of children in clinical trials. By 1998, strong advocacy by pediatric organizations resulted in the NIH creating a policy requiring the inclusion of children in NIH-supported clinical trials.[11] However, unlike the 1993 federal law on inclusion of "women and minorities," the child-focused NIH policy was not codified in statute and was not accompanied by any systematic reporting requirements or other effective mechanisms to ensure compliance.

In addition to advocacy efforts directed at the NIH, the pediatric community also focused attention on the FDA. Clinical trials of most drugs did not include children, leading to extensive off-label drug use with limited information extrapolated from adult studies. In 1968, Shirkey described the situation well when he referred to children as "therapeutic orphans."[12] A first attempt to address this orphan status was the FDA Modernization and Accountability Act of 1997, which granted sponsors an additional six months of market exclusivity in return for voluntarily performing FDA requested studies in children.[13] In 2002, the Best Pharmaceuticals for Children Act (BPCA, Public Law 107–109) reauthorized pediatric exclusivity and created the Office of Pediatric Therapeutics within the FDA.[14] Following in 2003, the Pediatric Research Equity Act (PREA, Public Law 108–155) allowed the FDA to require the study of a new drug or biologic in pediatric populations.[15] These acts required congressional reauthorization every 5 years, and sustained pediatric advocacy was necessary to ensure reauthorization. After a decade of effort, BPCA and PREA were made permanent in 2012. Currently, most new drugs that might have use in children are tested in one or more pediatric trials. As a result of BPCA and PREA, 996 drug labels have been changed with new pediatric information.[16] A timeline of major milestones in pediatric clinical research advocacy is shown in **Box 1**.

COUNTING CHILDREN IN CLINICAL RESEARCH: A PERSONAL JOURNEY OF ADVOCACY

The previous background and history have been provided because effective advocates need to know what has gone before, and the magnitude of the efforts that have extended across multiple generations. My personal (SCD) advocacy journey began later in my career when I became a member of the Committee on Pediatric Research (COPR) of the American Academy of Pediatrics (AAP) in 2003 (my coauthors contributed to all efforts and my personal journey). I brought to COPR the background of a pediatrician who had pursued a traditional academic path, training in neonatal nutrition and metabolism, setting up a laboratory and clinical research infrastructure,

Box 1	
Timeline of major milestones in pediatric clinical research advocacy	
1962	National Institute of Child Health and Human Development (NICHD) founded
1977	Food and Drug Administration (FDA)—General considerations for clinical evaluation of drugs in infants and children
1997	Food and Drug Administration Modernization Act (FDAMA)—6 additional months market exclusivity for pediatric studies
1998	National Institute of Health (NIH) policy requiring inclusion of children in clinical research
2002	Best Pharmaceuticals for Children Act (BPCA)
2003	Pediatric Research Equity Act (PREA)
2007	BPCA and PREA reauthorized
2012	BPCA and PREA made permanent
2016	21st Century Cures Act

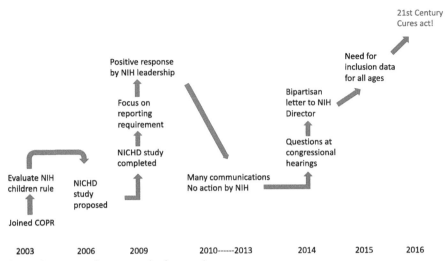

Fig. 1. Summary of a personal advocacy journey.

obtaining NIH funding, and conducting studies in neonates focusing on protein glucose and energy metabolism and requirements. All my work was human based, and I was a long-term member of the institutional review board. However, I had no experience in advocacy.

In addition to committee members appointed by the AAP Board of Directors, COPR also includes liaisons from most of the pediatric academic organizations. The director of the National Institutes of Child Health and Human Development (NICHD) also is a liaison to the committee. This makes the COPR an ideal forum to advocate for pediatric research at the federal level. In 2003, it had been 5 years since the NIH policy requiring the inclusion of children was implemented. The committee directed its attention to how well that policy was working. At the time, NIH defined children as less than 21 years old, leading to the concern that most children included in clinical trials were individuals between 18 and 21. There was no requirement for reporting how many children were included in clinical trials, unlike the mandatory reporting requirement for women and minorities.

In 2006, the NICHD launched a study to assess how well the inclusion of children rule was working within their NIH Institute. In 2009 the study was completed, and findings were shared with COPR, showing that even for projects funded by NICHD, many studies planned to exclude children and many others only planned to include those with ages between 18 and 21. Only plans for including children could be analyzed; the actual number of children studied could not be determined because there was no reporting requirement.

I was now Chair of COPR, and we decided to specifically focus our advocacy on requesting that the NIH add a reporting requirement (by age categories) for children. The necessity of the requirement was easily explained: (1) even the most basic question: "How many children were included in clinical trials at NIH?" could not be answered; (2) without these data, there was no ability to determine the efficacy of the NIH inclusion policy; and (3) there was already a requirement to report inclusion of "women and minorities" in clinical trials, so adding a requirement to report children would be a minimal burden for investigators.

Late in 2009, along with AAP leadership, I had the opportunity to meet with NIH leadership. I discussed the need for a reporting requirement for children, and the

---

Box 2
Advocacy Lessons Learned

Don't be intimidated
Advocacy can appear daunting from the outside. Your experience, education, and interests are everything you need to begin on an advocacy journey.

Work with experienced advocates
Find organizations with an advocacy infrastructure and a track record of success. These organizations will welcome you with open arms, and guide and support your journey. The American Academy of Pediatrics is a particularly good example, but there are many others.

Advocate for what you know and care about
Advocacy is most successful and sustainable when it comes from personal experience and passion. Authenticity counts for a lot.

Learn the history of previous advocacy efforts
Advocacy most often builds on previous efforts. Knowing what has gone before will make you a more effective advocate.

Understand the advocacy timeline
Recognize this is likely a long haul. Advocacy is rarely fast or linear. Persistence is necessary and progress often comes in spurts after long pauses.

Focus your ask
Ensuring children are included in clinical research has many complexities. Focusing on obtaining the data on inclusion had the advantage of being clear and easy to explain. It was also a necessary step to address the other complexities of inclusion. Whatever the advocacy issue, specificity and clarity are rewarded.

Be prepared for a relay race
Because of long advocacy timelines, the baton may need to pass multiple times. Work to make good exchanges.

Collect allies
Collecting allies is fundamental to advocacy. Be open to expected and unexpected allies. In the case of including children in clinical research, academic pediatric organizations were obvious and important allies. Based on the common interest of understanding inclusion in clinical research at all ages, aligning with advocates for the elderly was less obvious and perhaps even more important.

Sometimes policy is not enough
National Institute of Health policies on the inclusion of women and children in clinical research were not adequate. Pursuing legislation, although time-consuming and difficult, may be a final necessary step.

---

concept was very well received. A follow-up letter was sent by the AAP president to NIH leadership reiterating the need and rationale for the reporting requirement.

In 2010 the NIH established an internal task force to review its current policies and inclusion of women minorities and other populations in clinical research. The AAP reaffirmed the request for reporting requirements by age categories. Ultimately, there was no public report from the task force and no action on the reporting requirement for children was taken.

Over the next 2 years, despite multiple follow-up letters, conversations, and meetings with NIH personnel, no progress was made in instituting a reporting requirement for children. For reasons that remain opaque, it was apparent that the NIH did not have a plan or intent to institute the requirement.

In 2012, my term as chair of COPR ended. Although I stayed involved, COPR and the AAP continued the effort. Attention was now focused on Congress to encourage the NIH to institute the reporting requirement. In congressional hearings, NIH officials

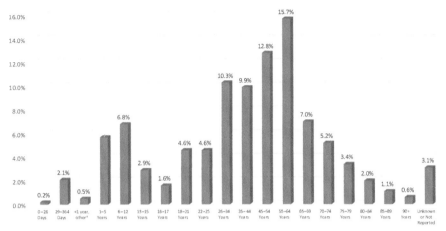

Fig. 2. Participant enrollment in NIH research by age group, FY 2021. [a]Includes ages reported in weeks, months, or years that are equivalent to less than 1 year. (*Source*: NIH, Extramural Nexus April2022. https://nexus.od.nih.gov/all/2022/04/11/fy-2021-data-on-age-at-enrollment-in-clinical-research-now-available-by-rcdc-category/.)

were asked about the number of children included in NIH-funded clinical trials, a question they could not answer. Discussions with members of Congress explaining the need for the reporting requirement were well received. In 2014, a bipartisan letter from 46 members of Congress was sent to the NIH director urging attention to the issue of the reporting requirement. This was ineffective, and it was clear that a congressional mandate was necessary.

As Congress was considering reporting requirements for children, it became apparent that there was also a need to understand how many older adults were included in NIH-sponsored clinical trials. Advocates for the elderly joined the effort as powerful allies. At the end of 2016, Congress passed, and the president signed the 21st Century Cures Act (PL 114–235).[17] Although this law addressed multiple aspects of research, it specifically required applicants for NIH funding to submit a plan for including individuals across the lifespan. It also required NIH to collect data on the inclusion of participants in clinical trials by age, culminating in over 10 years of advocacy efforts. A summary of my advocacy journey is shown in **Fig. 1**.

As an academician and clinician, I was certainly naive about advocacy at the federal level at the beginning of my journey. It seemed straightforward to identify a problem, propose an easily understood and logical solution, and expect action. The solution required only a minor modification of existing NIH policy and required no additional funding. Nevertheless, it literally required an act of Congress for implementation. A list of my lessons learned in advocacy is shown in **Box 2**.

CLINICAL RESEARCH INCLUSION ACROSS THE LIFESPAN: CURRENT STATE

After the passage of the 21st Century Cures Act, the NIH convened a workshop in 2017 focused on the inclusion of pediatric and older adult populations in clinical research, including clinical trials.[18] There were multiple recommendations from the workshop including these, directed at the culture of the scientific community:

Rather than trying to reduce the risk to vulnerable populations from research, the scientific community should consider how these populations might benefit from greater participation in such research, including the generation of efficacy data that

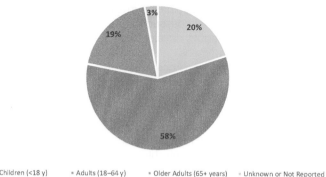

Fig. 3. Participant enrollment in NIH clinical research by broad age groups, FY21. (*Source*: NIH, Extramural Nexus April 2022. https://nexus.od.nih.gov/all/2022/04/11/fy-2021-data-on-age-at-enrollment-in-clinical-research-now-available-by-rcdc-category/.)

are applicable to them. Inclusion should be the default position, so that study design can focus on identifying ways to adopt responsible inclusion.

In response to these recommendations, the NIH made changes to the grant application and the review process to better ensure inclusion across the lifespan of clinical research.

Another recommendation from the workshop focused on the need for more detailed information regarding the age of individuals participating in clinical research. In response, the NIH now requires investigators to submit anonymized *individual*-level data on age and other demographics. Recently, the first data obtained on the ages of participants in NIH-sponsored clinical trials became available.[19] These data, for the NIH in total for FY 2021, are shown in **Figs. 2** and **3**. These are only 1 year of data, and these were obtained during the pandemic, so they may not be fully representative. Nevertheless, it appears that adolescents and older adults (>70 years) may be underrepresented. This will require continued attention as additional data become available, including comparisons across NIH Institutes.

CONTINUED ADVOCACY OPPORTUNITIES FOR INCLUSION

Now that data on inclusion are available from NIH, the pediatric community must carefully monitor this information to ensure inclusion and identify opportunities for improvement. In addition, although children are included in most drug trials, challenges remain for devices and diagnostic tests.[20] There remain significant barriers for pregnant women and across racial and ethnic groups to fully participate in clinical trials.[21–23] Continued and persistent advocacy is necessary to achieve full inclusion so that clinical research can provide the maximum benefit to the whole population. History tells us we must continue to speak up for children.

REFERENCES

1. Moon MR, Khin-Maung-Gyi F. The history and role of institutional review boards. Virtual Mentor 2009;11:311–21.

2. The belmont report: ethical principles and guidelines for the protection of human subjects of research. https://www.hhs.gov/ohrp/regulations-and-policy/belmont-report/read-the-belmont-report/index.html (Accessed July 7, 2022).

3. (ORWH) history of women's participation in clinical rearch. https://orwh.od.nih. gov/toolkit/recruitment/history (Accessed July 7, 2022).
4. FDA. Gender Studies in product development: historical overview. https://www. fda.gov/science-research/womens-health-research/gender-studies-product-development-historical-overview (Accessed July 7, 2022).
5. Kim ES, Menon V. Status of women in cardiovascular clinical trials. Arterioscler Thromb Vasc Biol 2009;29:279–83.
6. Merkatz RB. Inclusion of women in clinical trials: a historical overview of scientific, ethical, and legal issues. J Obstet Gynecol Neonatal Nurs 1998;27:78–84.
7. National Institutes of Health. NIH guidelines on the inclusion of women and minorities as subjects in clinical research. https://grants.nih.gov/grants/guide/notice-files/not94-100.html (Accessed July 7, 2022).
8. Denne SC, Hay WW Jr. Advocacy for research that benefits children: an obligation of pediatricians and pediatric investigators. JAMA Pediatr 2013;167:792–4.
9. NICHD History. https://www.nichd.nih.gov/about/history (Accessed July 7, 2022).
10. Children's Oncology Group. https://www.childrensoncologygroup.org/about (Accessed July 7, 2022).
11. NIH policy and guidelines on the inclusion of children as participants in research involving human subjects. https://grants.nih.gov/grants/guide/notice-files/not98-024.html (Accessed July 7, 2022).
12. Shirkey H. Therapeutic orphans. J Pediatr 1968;72:119–20.
13. FDA modernization act of 1997. https://www.govinfo.gov/content/pkg/PLAW-105publ115/pdf/PLAW-105publ115.pdf (Accessed July 7, 2022).
14. Best pharmaceuticals for children act. https://www.congress.gov/107/plaws/publ109/PLAW-107publ109.pdf (Accessed July 7, 2022).
15. Pediatric research equity act of 2003. https://www.congress.gov/108/plaws/publ155/PLAW-108publ155.pdf (Accessed July 7, 2022).
16. FDA 2022 pediatric labeling changes. https://www.fda.gov/science-research/pediatrics/pediatric-labeling-changes (Accessed July 7, 2022).
17. 21st century cures Act. https://www.congress.gov/114/plaws/publ255/PLAW-114publ255.pdf (Accessed July 7, 2022).
18. Bernard MA, Clayton JA, Lauer MS. Inclusion across the lifespan: NIH policy for clinical research. JAMA 2018;320:1535–6.
19. Lauer M. FY 2021 data on age at enrollment in clinical research. https://nexus.od. nih.gov/all/2022/04/11/fy-2021-data-on-age-at-enrollment-in-clinical-research-now-available-by-rcdc-category/ (Accessed July 7, 2022).
20. Caldwell CS, Denne SC. Rigorous and consistent evaluation of diagnostic tests in children: another unmet need. Pediatr Res 2020;88:524–5.
21. Denne SC. Including pregnant women in clinical research: time to overcome the barriers. Pediatr Res 2019;86:554–5.
22. Bibbins-Domingo K, Helman A, Dzau VJ. The imperative for diversity and inclusion in clinical trials and health research participation. JAMA 2022. https://doi.org/10.1001/jama.2022.9083.
23. Chen MS Jr, Lara PN, Dang JH, et al. Twenty years post-NIH Revitalization Act: enhancing minority participation in clinical trials (EMPaCT): laying the groundwork for improving minority clinical trial accrual: renewing the case for enhancing minority participation in cancer clinical trials. Cancer 2014;120(Suppl 7):1091–6.

Child Health Advocacy
The Journey to Antiracism

Joseph L. Wright, MD, MPH[a,b,c,]*, Tiffani J. Johnson, MD, MSc[d]

KEYWORDS

- Advocacy • Antiracism • Strategy

KEY POINTS

- The work of advancing equity and antiracism requires commitment, courage, humility, introspection, and resolve.
- Race is a social construct that reflects differential often inequitable lived experiences and should not be used as a biologic proxy.
- Pediatricians are well positioned to address structural and systemic inequities across the life course that contribute to health disparities.

INTRODUCTION

The last several years have seen accelerated activity and discourse directed at antiracism. Specifically following the 2020 murder of George Floyd, institutions across the country engaged in a range of introspective exercises and transparent reckonings examining their practices, policies, and history insofar as equity and racism is concerned. The authors of this article, both active protagonists in this domain, have been, and continue to be, part of ongoing national efforts and have learned much about the strategies and tactics necessary to initiate, engage, and sustain traction on the path to antiracism. Dr Johnson presents a comprehensive overview of racism, including definitions, historical context, its influence on children and adolescents and clearly establishes the case for antiracism advocacy. Dr Wright follows with reflections that intertwine personal experiences with leadership accountability enacted through a lens of equity and child health advocacy.

The authors have nothing to disclose.
[a] Department of Pediatrics, University of Maryland School of Medicine, Baltimore; [b] Department of Health Policy and Management, University of Maryland School of Public Health, College Park; [c] University of Maryland Medical System, 250 West Pratt Street, 24th Floor, Baltimore, MD 21201, USA; [d] Department of Emergency Medicine, University of California-Davis, 4150 V Street Suite 2100, Sacramento, CA 95817, USA
* Corresponding author. University of Maryland Medical System, 250 West Pratt Street, 24th Floor, Baltimore, MD 21201.
E-mail address: joseph.wright@umm.edu

Pediatr Clin N Am 70 (2023) 91–101
https://doi.org/10.1016/j.pcl.2022.09.014
0031-3955/23/© 2022 Elsevier Inc. All rights reserved.

OVERVIEW
A Brief Historical Context on Race and Racism in Medicine

Advocacy for antiracism in pediatrics begins with structural competency, including an understanding of key terms (**Box 1**) and the history of race and racism. Race is a social construct that has been closely tied with the concept of "white" as superior, serving as justification for colonization and the enslavement of African people. Medicine and science helped legitimize a narrative of Black genetic inferiority. For example, research measuring skulls across different races concluded that African people had smaller brain volumes and were, therefore, less intelligent than Caucasians, and dehumanized people of African descent arguing that each race was a separate species.[1] The term "drapetomania," was coined by a physician and defined as a mental health disorder among enslaved Black people with symptoms including the urge to run away, destroy property, disobey, talk back to enslavers, and refuse to work. Enslavers were encouraged to whip enslaved people and keep them in the position of submission that they were intended to occupy as a form of prevention and therapy.[2,3]

Such racist rhetoric of Black genetic inferiority proposed by the medical community served as justification to uphold slavery and white supremacy. The eugenics movement subsequently codified the disproportionate forced sterilization among minoritized groups to prevent the spread of violence, promiscuity, substance abuse, and intellectual inferiority.[4] The history of medicine also includes Black bodies being exploited in research.[5,6] These historic injustices must be viewed in light of modern times when there are several ways in which research continues to perpetuate racism and uphold structures of white supremacy. This includes both excluding racially diverse and socially marginalized groups in some research, whereas at other times exploiting and overrepresenting minoritized groups in research that does not require informed consent.

In 2020, the American Academy of Pediatrics (AAP) Board of Directors published the statement "Truth, Reconciliation, and Transformation: Continuing on the Path to Equity,"[7] detailing the discrimination faced by Dr Roland Boyd Scott and Dr Alonzo deGrate Smith who became the first Black members admitted into the AAP in 1945 6 years after their applications were rejected multiple times. The statement helps further highlight the sordid truth that our nation was built on a foundation of racism, and neither academic medicine more broadly nor the specialty of pediatrics are exceptions to this grim reality. The same Jim Crow Laws that segregated schools, water fountains, and buses in general society also served to segregate our academic organizations. This was true not only for providers from minoritized groups but also for our patients. It was not until 1965 that Medicare forced widespread desegregation in health care by threatening to withhold federal funding from hospitals who practiced racial discrimination in violation of the Civil Rights Act.[8]

This brief historical context helps illustrate the role that (pseudo)science and medicine played in constructing many of the negative associations held about racially minoritized groups created to uphold slavery and white supremacist ideology. This has been further reinforced in modern times through priming in media and popular culture.[9] Racist imagery has even been used in pharmaceutical marketing. For example, an advertisement in the Archives of General Psychiatry in 1974 featured an angry Black man shaking his fist, captioned "Assaultive and belligerent? Cooperation often begins with Haldol."[10]

Beyond the broader history around racism and medicine, it is important for practitioners to understand the demographics of the patient population that they serve, the history of racism in their community, and prior history of conflicts between their institution and the community that may affect patient and family trust in order to be

Box 1 Definition	
Term	**Definition**
Racism	A system of structuring opportunities and assigning value based on the social interpretation of how one looks (which is what we call "race") that unfairly disadvantages some individuals and communities and saps the strength of the whole society through the waste of human resources[a,b]
Personally mediated/ interpersonal racism	Occurs between individuals and can include explicit bias, implicit bias, racial discrimination, and microaggressions
Explicit bias	Conscious attitudes towards a person, group, or idea that can be self-reported
Implicit bias	Attitudes toward a person, group, or idea that we are not consciously aware of but can influence our behaviors
Racial discrimination	Unjust differential treatment based on race
Microaggressions	"The everyday verbal, nonverbal, and environmental slights, snubs, or insults, whether intentional or unintentional, which communicate hostile, derogatory or negative messages to target persons based solely upon their marginalized group membership"[c]
Institutional racism	Policies or practices within an organization (eg, hospitals, schools) that unfairly advantage white individuals and communities while unfairly disadvantaging racially minoritized groups
Minoritized	Social groups (eg, race, religion, sex, gender identity, sexual orientation) that are systematically devalued and unfairly disadvantaged in society. This devaluing includes how the group is represented and what resources they have access to. Although these groups have traditionally been referred to as *minorities*, replacing this language with the term *minoritized* better captures the forces that create the lower status in society. Furthermore, because people of color represent the global majority, it helps signal that a group's status is not necessarily related to their proportion of the population[d]
Structural racism	Local, state, and national policies, laws, and regulations that systematically create differential access to services and opportunities in society based on race
Antiracism	Identifying and confronting unearned power and unjust policies that uphold racism, whereas advocating for the equitable distribution of power and new policies rooted in justice[e]

[a]Jones, CP. Confronting institutionalized racism. Phylon. 2002; 50(1/2):7-22. [b]Johnson TJ. Antiracism, Black Lives Matter, and Critical Race Theory: The ABCs of promoting equity in pediatrics. Pediatric Annals. 2022; 51(3):e95-e106. [c]Sue DW, Capodilupo CM, Torino GC, Bucceri JM, Holder A, Nadal KLEsquilin M. Racial microaggressions in everyday life: implications for clinical practice. American Psychologist 2007;62(4):271-286. [d]Sensoy O and DiAngelo R. Is Everyone Really Equal?: An Introduction to Key Concepts in Social Justice Education, first edition. Teacher's College Press: New York, 2012, p. 5. [e]Kendi IX. How to be an antiracist. New York: One World, 2019.

effective advocates for antiracism. Providers should also examine and confront their personal biases. This can begin with taking the publicly available implicit association test, engaging in group discussions about insights gained, and applying evidence-informed bias reduction strategies (eg, perspective taking, stereotype replacement, individuation, exploring common identities, cross-cultural contact mindfulness, attention to talk time ratios).[11]

Children's Experiences of Racism

Taking social determinants of health lens, racism affects where children and adolescents live, play, and learn, how they are policed, as well as access to and experiences in the health-care system. For example, the discriminatory practice of redlining shaped the residential segregation that persists in neighborhoods today.[12] In modern times, minoritized groups continue to face discrimination in rental applications, mortgage lending, and the devaluation of housing based on owner and neighborhood demographics.[13–15] Persistent residential segregation also limits access to recreation and green spaces for minoritized communities. In the education setting, minoritized youth experience pervasive disparities in suspensions and expulsions, as well as enrollment in special education and advance placement classes. Policing has also become an important social determinant of health, with minoritized youth being overpoliced and underprotected.[16] In the health-care system, minoritized youth experience pervasive disparities in care and outcomes that are rooted in bias and institutionalized racism.

Impact of Racism on Health

Encountering racism across multiple aspects of one's lived experiences has adverse impacts on health and wellness. The most robust evidence exists for emotional/behavioral health outcomes, where individuals who report experiencing racism are more likely to experience anxiety, depression, and poor sleep.[17,18] There is also growing evidence of the impact of experiencing racism on the cardiovascular system, including higher risk of hypertension and myocardial infarction in adult populations.[19–21] In the endocrine system, experiences of racism are associated with larger waist circumferences, higher Body Mass Index, obesity, and diabetes.[22–24] We also see dysregulation of immune function and inflammatory response.[25,26] Racism is also associated with epigenetic changes linked with gene expression and accelerated aging.[27,28]

ADVOCACY PERSPECTIVES

Equipped with a greater understanding of racism and its impact on health and wellness, pediatric providers are better positioned to serve as advocates for antiracism. These perspectives (Joseph Wright's) are first-hand accounts presented through the story-telling vehicle of minivignettes, in and of itself an effective advocacy tool. The emphasis is on lessons learned, strategies and tactics used, with context framed largely through experiences related to leadership accountabilities in organized pediatrics.

Leaves and Roots

At the beginning of my term as a member of the American Academy of Pediatrics Board of Directors, I was introduced to an exercise known as leaves and roots that I have since adopted as a content icebreaker for presentations on equity and antiracism. Designed primarily as a networking activity to foster deeper connections with colleagues, the leaves on the figurative tree represent things that are readily visible such as hobbies, demographic information, distinguishable personal traits, things you do well, and so forth. The tree's roots, on however, reveal things that are not easily visible such as where you are from, values, important life events, things you may struggle with, and so forth. Applying the leaves and roots instrument to my personal journey as prelude to discussion about the importance of recognizing and respecting differential lived experiences has proven an effective tool in engaging audiences. It has been particularly effective in settings where there may be collegial or tacit familiarity with my background at the level of "leaves." Digging into the "roots," especially those which directly identify racism as an integral contributor to my and my family's lived experiences, both historical and contemporary, has become a powerful platform from which to launch discussion about bias, preconceived perceptions, and the need for personal introspection. Feedback regarding this exercise has been overwhelmingly positive with participants typically experiencing greater engagement efficacy with what can be challenging and difficult content to embrace. Notably, there have also been a very small number of responses citing the transparent and personalized discussion of the influence of racism as uncomfortable and perhaps even triggering. One respondent even suggested that a disclosure be issued at the beginning of the talk warning about the nature of the leaves and roots content.

Skewing to the Science

Antiracism advocacy can often feel disquieting and polarizing. I have presented such educational content in many a setting where I have seen participants literally get up and walk out of the room. Unfamiliarity with unvarnished truth about racism in our society and ignorance of the differential lived experiences of minoritized people, even when they are our patients, can breed discomfort. I am often challenged in sharing such knowledge by the comment "What does this have to do with me? I am not a racist." One of the questions I am frequently asked by fellow advocates is "How do we get our colleagues to listen; how do we capture their attention?"

A tactic that is certainly not unique to antiracism advocacy is skewing the discourse to the evidence. Especially for provider audiences, appealing to the inner scientist at the core of our training is a way to objectively communicate, sometimes, difficult and cognitively dissonant concepts. Moreover, there is certainly no dearth of evidence, ranging from basic science to clinical investigations, associated with the pervasive impact of structural inequities, institutional bias and discrimination, and societal racism on children and adolescents.[11,29] Particularly compelling is the emerging literature on the intergenerational transmission of historically mediated racism, which is right in the scientific wheelhouse for pediatricians steeped in the core understanding of the life course perspective of disease manifestation.[30–33]

A small evidence-informed convenience sample of disparities in plain sight that stem from structural, institutional, and systemic inequities include the following:

- Environmental injustice and disproportionate toxic exposures borne by marginalized communities today because of racist housing practices associated with redlining.[34] Beginning in the 1930s, the federal Home Owners' Loan Corporation marked areas across the United States as unworthy of loans because of an "infiltration of foreign-born, Negro, or lower grade population," and shaded them in red.[35] Despite being outlawed more than a half-century ago, redlining continues to affect people who live in neighborhoods that government mortgage officers shunned for 30 years. Redlining's echo is a profound and pervasive example of systematic racism and, incidently, lives prominently among my own leaves and roots.
- Perceptions of physiologic differences based solely on racial phenotypes. A 2016 study of white medical students and residents demonstrated that endorsement of false beliefs about the way in which Black people experience pain was

associated with lower pain score assessments and inaccurate treatment recommendations for Black patients compared with White patients in mock clinical scenarios.[36,37] Several recent studies have demonstrated that African American children with appendicitis and long bone fractures, respectively, receive opioid analgesia significantly less frequently than white patients and are less likely to achieve optimal pain reduction.[38–40]

- Kernicterus in Black newborns. Black babies are disproportionately represented in kernicterus databases at 25% despite making up 14% of the overall population of newborns.[41] Missed or delayed recognition of the acute hemolysis associated with glucose-6-phosphate dehydrogenase (G6PD) deficiency has been implicated among the root causes of this irreversible condition. Yet, until very recently the clinical practice guideline (CPG) on Management of Neonatal Hyperbilirubinemia in the Newborn Infant, originally published by the AAP in 2004, actually downgraded the algorithmic risk of severe hyperbilirubinemia in newborns race-assigned as Black obviating the urgency for aggressive diagnostic workup.[42] The revised CPG published in 2022 has addressed this issue by striking the race/ethnicity terms from among the independent variables included in assessing risk for severe hyperbilirubinemia, and emphasizing the critical importance of probing ancestry as a critical component of the decision-making process in the assessment of jaundice. Pediatricians need to understand the underlying biology of G6PD and the relevance of its geographic distribution around the world.[43,44]

Skewing to the science is critical in written communication as well. Lack of fundamental knowledge of the sordid history of racism in this country, much of which has been surreptitiously hidden, can sow seeds of doubt for readers who may be trying to ascend a learning curve and are confronted with ugly, unbelievable truth. Therefore, it is important to make every effort to identify multiple primary sources, to be expansive in capturing relevant interdisciplinary studies from diverse platforms, and to explicitly cite and call out the pseudoscience used to justify slavery and that has supported the persistence of discriminatory beliefs and practices. For instance, a recently published AAP policy statement, "Eliminating Race-Based Medicine," although less than 4000 words was supported by more than 100 references ranging during a 250-year period in an explicit effort to bolster the recommended actions with unequivocal and well-cited truth.[45]

Flooding the Field

We all bring unique perspectives to this work influenced by our personal circumstances, longitudinal exposures and differential lived experiences. Institutions and organizations, similarly, are on varying trajectories and glidepaths in actualizing antiracism activity. For instance, the partner organizations that comprise the Pediatric Academic Societies (PAS), the Academic Pediatric Association, the AA P, the American Pediatric Society, and the Society for Pediatric Research have all taken notable steps over the last several years in the advancement of equity, diversity, and inclusion and promotion of antiracism agendas.[7,46–48] However, the reality is, and will be for quite some time, that as advocates, activists, participants, and leaders, we are all in different places on our individual and collective antiracism journeys. This study can feel positively disruptive and progressive, while at the same time feel frustratingly bogged down in polarized inertia. It is therefore incumbent on all of us to accept and embrace that antiracism advocacy is necessarily iterative and incremental work. Not unlike the first several steps on the spiraling yellow brick road in the Wizard of Oz, the work of advancing an antiracism agenda requires repetition, assurance, reassurance, validation, education, reeducation, and may think like little progress is being made. However, it is deliberate understanding of this iterative approach that will ultimately begin to move the needle and advance discourse from just preaching to the choir to engaging whole congregations.

With this strategy in mind, tactically, at the 2022 PAS meeting, several academic institution-based advocates and organized medicine leaders collaborated to "flood the field" with multiple antiracism focused plenary session submissions. Ranging from state-of-the-science plenaries to high-powered panel discussions to provocative hot topic sessions, leaders from all 4 PAS partner organizations intentionally committed significant conference time and space to antiracism content. The engagement and exchange with conference attendees, especially those in early career, was indeed iterative, as intended and laid groundwork for broader ongoing efforts.

Engaging Editors

The biology of adversity is a complex milieu anchored by systemic and structural inequities that play out over the life course. The pediatric community understands this well and is uniquely positioned to address the attendant interventional challenges. Therefore, in academic and organized pediatrics, the immediate task is to

- Recognize racism in all its forms,
- Call it explicitly by name,
- Declaratively oppose it, and
- Most importantly, unequivocally enact commitment and resolve to actively replace it.[49]

The last 5 years across the PAS has seen a sea change in openly "calling the question" on racism. As recently as 2017, in a commentary authored by leadership representatives of several of the PAS partner and affiliate organizations and copublished in 3 of the organizations' academic journals, "The Road to Tolerance and Understanding" danced around the issue without actually referencing the term "racism" anywhere in the article.[50-52] In 2019, the AAP policy statement, "The Impact of Racism on Child and Adolescent Health" was the first such statement published in the peer-reviewed literature by a major medical society to not only directly name racism but also highlight its eradication as a matter of organizational policy.[29] Moreover in 2020, the APS Committee on Diversity, Inclusion and Equity authored a series of commentaries entitled the APS Racism Series published on the editorial pages of *Pediatric Research* that not only called the question but also broadened the scientific dialogue through a series of companion town hall discussions that were open to all members of the pediatric community.[53-56] The last 2 years have seen the editorial boards of pediatric and other journals open platforms for commentary and discussion focused on equity issues and eliciting viewpoints from an increasingly diverse pool of authors, advocates and thought leaders.[57-60] This proactive engagement with journal editors and editorial boards is a powerful tactic in order to more broadly disseminate differential perspectives across an array of audiences thus introducing more folks to active antiracism concepts.

Withering and Weathering

Authentic commitment to antiracism advocacy can feel withering, especially in the current political and social climate. There is so much to be done and the stark realization that this study is both transformational and generational can feel daunting. Further, the burden of carrying the antiracism mantle is often disproportionately borne by those underrepresented in medicine, who must reconcile institutional responsibilities with personally operating in challenging professional environments. The consequences of the so-called minority tax[61,62] can not only feel withering on a daily basis but can also be deleterious to personal physical and mental health, and professional advancement.[63] The relationship of differential allostatic load bearing by American descendants of slavery has been linked to the concept of physiologic weathering, of which shortened telomeres in African American men have been posited as a measurable biomarker.[32,64,65] Additionally, yes, I do worry about the length of my telomeres and those of my sons.

The flip side of the withering-weathering concern, however, is that assuredly there is a personal resilience derived from commitment to this study and to focusing on child health advocacy in general. I am particularly excited at the prospect of continued discovery in the domain of epigenetics. We are beginning to understand that the epigenome is neuro-developmentally dynamic[66,67] and that identifying protective mechanisms conferred by adverse exposures, including those associated with racism, is possible. So, although the journey to antiracism is definitely arduous, sobering, and oft-times painful, I think a cautious optimism that through ongoing advocacy, education and discovery that sustained progress can be achieved in my lifetime. Racism and racist principles have been both blatantly and surreptitiously embedded in the foundational fabric of the United States for more than 400 years; they will not be unwound overnight.

CLINICS CARE POINTS

- Racism as a component of children's lived experiences can have deleterious developmental, epigenetic, and physiologic impacts.
- Racial socialization, or the process by which children learn to navigate race issues, is an important element of anticipatory guidance and should be incorporated into longitudinal care.
- Practice guidelines must be scrutinized for the inappropriate inclusion of race assignment as a corrective, risk-adjusting, or dichotomizing variable in the clinical decision-making process.

REFERENCES

1. Mitchell PW. The fault in his seeds: lost notes to the case of bias in Samuel George Morton's cranial race science. PLoS Biol 2018;16(10):e2007008.
2. Suite DH, La Bril R, Primm A, et al. Beyond misdiagnosis, misunderstanding and mistrust: relevance of the historical perspective in the medical and mental health treatment of people of color. J Natl Med Assoc 2007;99(8):879.
3. Cartwright SA. Report on the diseases and physical peculiarities of the negro race. N Orleans Med Surg J 1851;VII:692–713.
4. Allen GE. Eugenics and modern biology: critiques of eugenics, 1910–1945. Ann Hum Genet 2011;75(3):314–25.
5. Galán CA, Bekele B, Boness C, et al. A call to action for an antiracist clinical science. J Clin Child Adolesc Psychol 2021;50(1):12–57.
6. Hardeman RR. Examining racism in health services research: a disciplinary self-critique. Health Serv Res 2020;55(Suppl 2):777.
7. American Academy of Pediatrics Board of Directors. Truth, reconciliation, and transformation: continuing on the path to equity. Pediatrics 2020;146(3). e2020019794.
8. Gordon E. Medicare and the desegregation of health care. WHYY; 2018. Available at: https://whyy.org/segments/medicare-desegregation-health-care/. Accessed June 7, 2022.

9. Sonnett J, Johnson KA, Dolan MK. Priming implicit racism in television news: visual and verbal limitations on diversity. Sociological Forum 2015;30(2):328–47.

10. Advertisement for haldol. Arch Gen Psychiatry 1974;31(5):732–3.

11. Johnson TJ. Racial bias and its impact on children and adolescents. Pediatr Clin North Am 2020;67(2):425–36.

12. Hiller AE. Redlining and the home owners' loan corporation. J Urban Hist 2003; 29(4):394–420.

13. Rosen E, Garboden PME, Cossyleon JE. Racial discrimination in housing: how landlords use algorithms and home visits to screen tenants. Am Sociol Rev 2021;86(5):787–822.

14. Hanson A, Hawley Z, Martin H, et al. Discrimination in mortgage lending: Evidence from a correspondence experiment. J Urban Econ 2016;92:48–65.

15. Howell J, Korver-Glenn E. Neighborhoods, race, and the twenty-first-century housing appraisal industry. Sociol Race Ethn 2018;4(4):473–90.

16. Johnson TJ, Wright JL. Executions and police conflicts involving children, adolescents and young adults. Pediatr Clin 2021;68(2):465–87.

17. Priest N, Paradies Y, Trenerry B, et al. A systematic review of studies examining the relationship between reported racism and health and wellbeing for children and young people. Social Sci Med 2013;95:115–27.

18. Slopen N, Lewis TT, Williams DR. Discrimination and sleep: a systematic review. Sleep Med 2016;18:88–95.

19. Dolezsar CM, McGrath JJ, Herzig AJM, et al. Perceived racial discrimination and hypertension: a comprehensive systematic review. Health Psychol 2014;33(1): 20–34.

20. Lukachko A, Hatzenbuehler ML, Keyes KM. Structural racism and myocardial infarction in the United States. Social Sci Med 2014;103:42–50.

21. Lee AK, Corneille MA, Hall NM, et al. The stressors of being young and black: cardiovascular health and Black young adults. Psychol Health 2016;31(5): 578–91.

22. Bacon KL, Stuver SO, Cozier YC, et al. Perceived racism and incident diabetes in the Black Women's Health Study. Diabetologia 2017;60(11):2221–5.

23. Dougherty GB, Golden SH, Gross AL, et al. Measuring structural racism and its association with BMI. Am J Prev Med 2020;59(4):530–7.

24. Stepanikova I, Baker EH, Simoni ZR, et al. The role of perceived discrimination in obesity among African Americans. Am J Prev Med 2017;52(1):S77–85.

25. Brody GH, Yu T, Miller GE, et al. Discrimination, racial identity, and cytokine levels among African-American adolescents. J Adolesc Health 2015;56(5):496–501.

26. Cuevas Adolfo G, Ong AD, Carvalho K, et al. Discrimination and systemic inflammation: A critical review and synthesis. Brain Behav Immun 2020;89:465–79.

27. de Mendoza VB, Huang Y, Crusto CA, et al. Perceived racial discrimination and DNA methylation among African American women in the InterGEN study. Biol Res Nurs 2018;20(2):145–52.

28. Chae DH, Nuru-Jeter AM, Adler NE, et al. Discrimination, racial bias, and telomere length in African-American men. Am J Prev Med 2014;46(2):103–11.

29. Trent M, Dooley DG, Douge J. American academy of pediatrics, section on adolescent health, council on community pediatrics; committee on adolescence. The impact of racism on child and adolescent health. Pediatrics 2019;144(2): e20191765.

30. Dias BG, Ressler KJ. Parental olfactory experience influences behavior and neural structure in subsequent generations. Nat Neurosci 2014;17(1):89–96.

31. Heard-Garris NJ, Cale M, Camaj L, et al. Transmitting trauma: a systematic review of vicarious racism and child health. Soc Sci Med 2018;199:230–40.

32. Johnstone SE, Baylin SB. Stress and the epigenetic landscape: a link to the pathobiology of human diseases? Nat Rev Genet 2010;11(11):806–12.

33. Bird A. Perceptions of epigenetics. Nature 2007;447(7143):396–8.

34. Lane HM, Morello-Frosch R, Marshall JD, et al. Historical redlining is associated with present-day air pollution disparities in U.S. cities. Environ Sci Technol Lett 2022;9(4):345–50.

35. Fears D. Redlining means 45 million Americans are breathing dirtier air 50 years after it ended. Washington Post. 2022. Available at: https://www.washingtonpost.com/climate-environment/2022/03/09/redlining-pollution-environmental-justice/. Accessed July 10, 2022.

36. Hoffman KM, Trawalter S, Axt JR, et al. Racial bias in pain assessment and treatment recommendations, and false beliefs about biological differences between blacks and whites. Proc Natl Acad Sci U S A 2016;113(16):4296–301.

37. Villarosa L. Myths about physical racial differences were used to justify slavery—and are still believed by doctors today. New York Times. 2019. Available at: https://www.nytimes.com/interactive/2019/08/14/magazine/racial-differences-doctors.html. Accessed January 30, 2022.

38. Goyal MK, Kuppermann N, Cleary SD, et al. Racial disparities in pain management of children with appendicitis in emergency departments. JAMA Pediatr 2015;169:996–1002.

39. Goyal MK, Johnson TJ, Chamberlain JM, et al, Pediatric Emergency Care Applied Research Network (PECARN). Racial and ethnic differences in emergency department pain management of children with fractures. Pediatrics 2020;145(5):e20193370.

40. Goyal MK, Drendel AL, Chamberlain JM, et al. Pediatric Emergency Care Applied Research Network (PECARN) Registry Study Group. Racial/Ethnic differences in ED opioid prescriptions for long bone fractures: trends over time. Pediatrics 2021;148(5). e2021052481.

41. Okolie F, South-Paul JE, Watchko JF. Combating the hidden health disparity of kernicterus in Black infants: a review. JAMA Pediatr 2020 Dec 1;174(12): 1199–205.

42. Maisels MJ, Baltz RD, Bhutani VK, et al. Management of hyperbilirubinemia in the newborn infant 35 or more weeks of gestation. Pediatrics 2004;114:297–316 [Erratum in Pediatrics. 2004;2114(2004):1138].

43. Kemper AR, Newman TB, Slaughter JL, et al. Clinical practice guideline revision: management of hyperbilirubinemia in the newborn infant 35 or more weeks of gestation. Pediatrics 2022;150(3):e2022058859.

44. Wright JL, Trent ME. Applying an equity lens to clinical practice guidelines: getting out of the gate. Pediatrics 2022;150(3):e2022058918.

45. Wright JL, Davis WS, Joseph MM, et al. Eliminating race-based medicine. Pediatrics 2022;150(1). e2022057998.

46. Academic Pediatric Association. Diversity, inclusion and equity statements. Available at: https://www.academicpeds.org/announcements/academic-pediatric-association-releases-diversity-inclusion-and-equity-statements/. Accessed June 13, 2022.

47. Abman SH, Bogue CW, Baker S, et al, American Pediatric Society (APS). Racism and social injustice as determinants of child health: the American Pediatric Society issue of the year. Pediatr Res 2020;88(5):691–3.

48. Abman SH, Armstrong S, Baker S, et al. The American Pediatric Society and Society for Pediatric Research joint statement against racism and social injustice. Pediatr Res 2022 Jan;91(1):264.

49. Ward JV. The skin we're in: teaching our teens to be emotional strong, socially smart, and spiritually connected. New York, NY: Free Press; 2002.

50. Szilagyi PG, Dreyer BP, Fuentes-Afflick E, et al. The road to tolerance and understanding. Acad Pediatr 2017 Jul;17(5):459–61.

51. Szilagyi PG, Dreyer BP, Fuentes-Afflick E, et al. The road to tolerance and understanding. Pediatrics 2017 Jun;139(6):e20170741.

52. Szilagyi PG, Dreyer BP, Fuentes-Afflick E, et al. The road to tolerance and understanding. J Adolesc Health 2017;60(6):631–3.

53. Abman SH. Holistic Promotion of Scholarship and Advancement" APS racism series: at the intersection of equity, science, and social justice. Pediatr Res 2020; 88(5):694–5.

54. Wright JL, Jarvis JN, Pachter LM, et al. Racism as a Public Health Issue" APS Racism Series: at the Intersection of Equity, Science and Social Justice. Pediatr Res 2020;88(5):696–8.

55. Walker-Harding LR, Bogue CW, Hendricks-Munoz KD, et al. Challenges and opportunities in academic medicine" APS racism series: at the intersection of equity, science, and social justice. Pediatr Res 2020;88(5):699–701.

56. Pursley DM, Coyne-Beasley TD, Freed GL, et al. Organizational solutions: calling the question" APS racism series: at the intersection of equity, science and social justice. Pediatr Res 2020;88(5):702–3.

57. Equity, diversity and inclusion feature. Available at: https://publications.aap.org/pediatrics/pages/author-instructions?autologincheck=redirected#diversity_equity_inclusion. Accessed June 29, 2022.

58. Johnson TJ. Intersection of bias, structural racism, and social determinants with health care inequities. Pediatrics 2020;146(2). e2020003657.

59. Raphael JL, Oyeku SO. Implicit bias in pediatrics: an emerging focus in health equity research. Pediatrics 2020;145(5):e20200512.

60. Wright JL, Freed GL, Hendricks-Muñoz KD, et al, Committee on Diversity, Inclusion and Equity on behalf of the American Pediatric Society. Achieving equity through science and integrity: dismantling race-based medicine. Pediatr Res 2022;91(7):1641–4.

61. Cyrus KD. A piece of my mind: medical education and the minority tax. JAMA 2017;317(18):1833–4.

62. Rodríguez JE, Campbell KM, Pololi LH. Addressing disparities in academic medicine: what of the minority tax? BMC Med Educ 2015;15:6.

63. Wright JL, Golden WC. See it to be it: diversity and inclusion in academic pediatrics starts at the top. Pediatrics 2022;150:e2022057435.

64. Geronimus AT, Hicken M, Keene D, et al. Weathering" and age patterns of allostatic load scores among blacks and whites in the United States. Am J Public Health 2006;96(5):826–33.

65. Simons RL, Lei MK, Klopack E, et al. Racial discrimination, inflammation, and chronic illness among African American women at midlife: support for the weathering perspective. J Racial Ethn Health Dispar 2021;8(2):339–49.

66. Kolb B, Harker A, Gibb R. Principles of plasticity in the developing brain. Dev Med Child Neurol 2017;59(12):1218–23.

67. Smeeth D, Beck S, Karam EG, et al. The role of epigenetics in psychological resilience. Lancet Psychiatry 2021;8(7):620–9.

Advocacy for Unaccompanied Migrant Children in US Detention

Paul H. Wise, MD, MPH

KEYWORDS

- Immigrant children • Advocacy • Immigration policy • Immigration detention

KEY POINTS

- An unprecedented number of unaccompanied migrant children are being apprehended on the US –Mexican border.
- Customs and Border Protection, a component of the Department of Homeland Security, and the Office of Refugee Resettlement, a unit within the Department of Health and Human Services, have primary responsibility for the custodial care and processing of unaccompanied migrant children.
- There are major advocacy opportunities to improve custodial conditions and processing, but these may depend on system reforms requiring enhanced coordination between agencies.
- Advocacy efforts, however, will need to navigate a complex policy environment in which a concern for children must contend with a divisive political discourse surrounding immigration policy.

Highly restrictive public sentiment toward immigration is not new in the United States.[1] What is new is how this restrictive US posture should apply to the unprecedented numbers of children crossing the border without a parent or legal guardian. In 2019, Linton and colleagues published in this journal an excellent review of the critical issues facing migrant children and their families once they enter the United States.[2] Earlier discussions have also presented essential information regarding systems of migrant child detention.[3,4] The current article seeks to complement this earlier work by identifying the current and emerging challenges and opportunities for advocacy dedicated to ensuring just and high-quality custodial care for unaccompanied migrant children who are held in US immigration detention.

Freeman Spogli Institute for International Studies, Stanford University, Encina Commons, Room 226, Stanford, CA 94305, USA
E-mail address: pwise@stanford.edu

Pediatr Clin N Am 70 (2023) 103–116
https://doi.org/10.1016/j.pcl.2022.09.006
0031-3955/23/© 2022 Published by Elsevier Inc.

pediatric.theclinics.com

THE CHALLENGE

Unaccompanied alien children (UACs) are defined in US statute as children who (1) lack lawful immigration status in the United States; (2) are under the age of 18; and (3) are without either a parent or legal guardian in the United States or a parent or legal guardian in the United States who is available to provide care and physical custody.[5] An alien is an individual who is not a US citizen or national.

Although many official documents use the term UAC, this discussion uses the term unaccompanied children (UCs). Children who are apprehended in the care of a trusted adult other than a parent or legal guardian, such as a grandmother or adult sibling, are currently considered UCs and processed as if they were encountered traveling on their own.

The number of UCs entering detention on the US southern border has reached unprecedented levels. During the 2000s, the annual number of UCs apprehended at the border ranged between 4,800 and 8,200. However, beginning in 2011, this figure began to increase, reaching almost 70,000 by 2014, and a level that overwhelmed existing detention capabilities for minors and first raised the specter of a humanitarian crisis involving children at the border.[6] At first considered a temporary phenomenon, these relatively high figures persisted until 2020 when the COVID-19 pandemic reduced migrant flows significantly. However, beginning in March 2021, the number of UCs apprehended at the border began to increase dramatically, rising to almost 19,000 for the month of July alone and ultimately totaling approximately 147,000 for the fiscal year (October–September), by far the highest in history[7] (**Fig. 1**). This trend has continued as the figure for 2022 is running 25% higher than the comparable period for 2021. Although the demographic distribution of UCs continues to evolve, most are leaving their home communities in the Northern Triangle countries of Central America: Guatemala, Honduras, and El Salvador.

Nevertheless, there has been a growing portion of UCs from Haiti, Venezuela, and Nicaragua, and other parts of the world.[7]

Advocacy requires a deep understanding of the forces driving UC migration to the US border, forces that are both varied and highly interactive. There has been a traditional tendency to dichotomize the reasons for migration into "voluntary" motivations, usually rooted in economic incentives, and "forced" motivations, most commonly associated with political persecution or a direct threat of violence. Although this dichotomization may conform to bureaucratic or legal distinctions in assessing immigration claims, empirical evidence suggests that from many areas of the world,

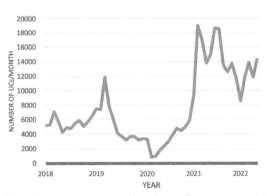

Fig. 1. Customs and border protection apprehensions of unaccompanied children, 2018 to 2022 (through May).

including the Northern Triangle of Central America and Haiti, decisions to migrate almost always involve a blurred combination of economic aspirations and the pursuit of refuge from extreme violence.[8,9] Guatemala, Honduras, El Salvador, and Haiti are among the poorest countries in the Western Hemisphere.[10] Social mobility has stagnated or declined.[11] Child malnutrition and stunted growth are all too common and child mortality and other adverse outcomes remain tragically elevated.[12] It is also important to recognize that many of these areas are experiencing the ravages of climate change. Severe hurricanes have beleaguered the Caribbean and Central America in recent years and serious agricultural plagues have reduced harvests in ways that have decimated the incomes of rural farmers and laborers.[13] These areas have also witnessed a serious deterioration in physical security with violent death rates that are second only to those found in active combat zones, such as Syria and Ukraine. Indeed, the levels of violent death, sexual assault, kidnapping, and general corruption in the Northern Triangle of Central America are among the highest in the world.[14,15] Together, this landscape of material deprivation, blunted opportunity, and desperate insecurity has generated the powerful yet inextricably interwoven origins of mass migration to the United States.

CURRENT DETENTION SYSTEMS FOR UNACCOMPANIED CHILDREN

Placing children in detention of any kind requires justification. The primary reason that unaccompanied migrant children are placed into detention by the US government is that an appropriate adult must be identified to assume responsibility for the child's care before any release or removal to a home country. Once apprehended, therefore, unaccompanied minors are placed in a federal system designed to provide custodial care until such a responsible adult can be identified. There is also a law enforcement requirement associated with detention. Beyond the issues of national sovereignty and border integrity, there is a need to ensure that children are not traveling with adults that pose a risk[16] or are being trafficked, a problem that remains of primary concern.[17–19] Adolescents are also screened for serious criminal histories.[5]

The detention of unaccompanied migrant children, therefore, has been justified on both child welfare and security grounds. However, these objectives are addressed by a system of custodial care primarily involving two federal agencies with vastly different missions, capabilities, and histories. It is useful for advocacy, therefore, to briefly review the structure of current custodial systems for UCs with an emphasis on those procedures and custodial practices that demand urgent scrutiny.

Customs and Border Protection

Migrant children usually make their first contact with the US government when they encounter agents or officers of Customs and Border Protection (CBP) soon after crossing the border. Most of the migrant children are apprehended by the Border Patrol (BP), a component agency of CBP.[20] BP is responsible for policing the border between formal ports of entry, such as airports or international bridges. A relatively small number of migrant children are brought into custody by the Office of Field Operations of CBP, which is responsible for crossings at ports of entry.[5]

BP has divided the US–Mexican border into nine sectors: San Diego, El Centro, Yuma, Tucson, El Paso, Big Bend, Del Rio, Laredo, and the Rio Grande Valley, traditionally the busiest sector for UC apprehensions. Each sector operates a number of field stations which are generally used for detaining and processing migrants. Built primarily to hold adults, these stations are usually composed of hard-walled cells that may be kept at cool temperatures and dubbed "hieleras" ("iceboxes").[21] Most sectors have constructed new facilities or designated selected stations as Centralized Processing Centers which provide enhanced care for children and families. These enhancements include around the clock medical teams,[22] supplies of child necessities, such as diapers, baby foods, and child-sized clothing, and the placement of contracted "caregivers" who help provide direct care for young UCs and assist with showering and other hygiene essentials.[23] COVID-19 procedures have evolved over the course of the pandemic, with testing and isolation on entry to BP facilities instituted in 2022. Overcrowding has plagued some BP sectors, and times in custody have been protracted intermittently. Although custodial care in BP facilities has generally improved since 2019, monitoring authorities and any legal advocates remain vigilant regarding compliance with requisite standards and complaints of inadequate conditions, including poor food, irregular access to showers or medical care, and mistreatment by BP agents and contracted guards.[24,25]

Office of Refugee Resettlement

Once UCs are processed by BP, they are transferred to the care of the Office of Refugee Resettlement (ORR) (**Fig. 2**). Unlike BP, ORR is not a law enforcement agency but rather a unit within the Department of Health and Human Services with the explicit objective of providing custodial care that incorporates the "best child welfare practices in the least restrictive settings that are in the best interest of the child."[5,26] Custodial services in ORR care are far more extensive than those in CBP facilities and include educational, medical, mental health, and recreational programs.[26] Traditionally, ORR has relied on licensed shelters or foster families and is responsible for vetting the safety and appropriateness of households expected to receive the child upon release from government custody. Most of the children are released to a vetted sponsor, usually a parent or close relative already residing in the United States.[5]

In early 2021, an unprecedented increase in UC apprehensions overwhelmed the capacities of the federal custodial system responsible for UC care, a challenge exacerbated by occupancy reductions required by COVID-19 restrictions. The inability to transfer children to ORR custody created extreme overcrowding in BP facilities, a situation that generated unacceptable custodial conditions and risks to child safety and well-being.[27]

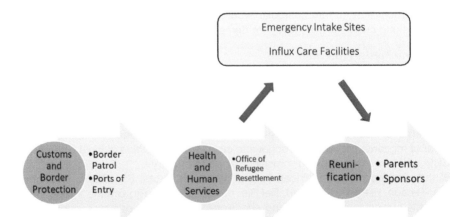

Fig. 2. US federal agencies comprising system of custodial care for unaccompanied migrant children. including Emergency Intake Sites and Influx Care Facilities.

In response, ORR established a new type of facility, the Emergency Intake Site (EIS), designed to quickly enhance ORRs custodial capacity and reduce the overcrowding in BP facilities.

Working closely with the Federal Emergency Management Agency, ORR opened 14 EISs in March and April of 2021, most using convention centers (which were vacant due to pandemic restrictions on large gatherings), "man camps" designed to house oil field workers, and a large newly erected, soft-sided tent facility at Ft. Bliss, near El Paso, Texas.[28]

The custodial standards at the EISs were far less comprehensive than those for licensed shelters, explicitly "designed for mass care with basic standards to meet immediate sheltering needs of unaccompanied children."[29] Although the EISs did substantially reduce the number of children in BP custody, the quality of care they provided raised serious concerns. By the spring of 2022, only the EISs at Pecos, Texas, and at Ft. Bliss remain operational. ORR has enhanced services at the EISs to reach those of what has been termed, an Influx Care Facility (ICF).[26] The transition of the two EISs to ICFs would provide three facilities with which ORR could respond to major increases in UC apprehensions on the border. Despite these substantial improvements in custodial conditions and family reunification processing, there remains an imperative to place children in licensed ORR facilities with the full range of custodial services.[28,30]

SPECIAL ADVOCACY CONSIDERATIONS

This article is premised on the contention that advocacy to improve the treatment for migrant children in US detention has a unique character, with elements of policy and public discourse that are not only distinctive but also strategic in the struggle for remedial reform. These distinct attributes are best articulated by an illustrative case: the Trump administration's child separation policy and the advocacy initiatives that opposed it.

CASE: Zero Tolerance Policy and Family Separation at the Border

On May 7, 2018, then-Attorney General Jeff Sessions announced a new policy to criminally prosecute all migrants apprehended entering the United States without authorization. Under this new mandate, dubbed the "Zero Tolerance" policy, all such apprehended migrants would be referred to the Department of Justice for criminal prosecution. No exceptions were made for migrants seeking asylum or for parents traveling with minor children, a decision that would necessarily result in immediate family separations.[31] This new policy was widely hailed by Trump administration officials and immigration enforcement advocates as the kind of strong measure that was necessary to discourage the increasing number of migrants seeking asylum at the US southern border. The announcement was accompanied by a major media blitz extolling the "game-changing" impact of this aggressive new policy.[32]

Yet, within 6 weeks of its announced implementation, the Zero Tolerance policy was dead. This dramatic reversal not only represents an example of a tragically bungled public initiative but also of a highly effective advocacy response that drew support from constituencies that cut across deep political and cultural lines. The policy was framed as a law enforcement strategy designed to deter unauthorized migrants from entering the United States. However, its reception among the American people was far more related to what it did to families, and more specifically, to children. Under the Zero Tolerance policy, the criminal prosecution of migrant parents required that they be detained in a federal criminal facility where children are not permitted. As a consequence, Zero Tolerance procedures resulted in family separation; parents were to be transferred to jail and children sent to ORR shelters as newly declared UCs.

The inherent linkage of Zero Tolerance to family separation set in motion a furious public debate. There was an immediate outcry from immigrant rights advocates. However, there was also a much broader societal unease with the growing realization that the government would use family separation as a deterrent to immigration. The public reception of the policy was made even more turbulent by the incoherence of the administration's defense of the family separation imperative.[33] Early on, senior national security officials admitted that family separation was not just a byproduct of the criminal prosecution of all adults but an explicit objective that was deemed necessary for aggressive deterrence.[34] Other administration leaders stated that family separation was a regrettable byproduct of the criminalization of unauthorized cross-border entry. Still others suggested that they had not known that Zero Tolerance would result in family separation, a claim of historic disingenuousness.[32,35]

Soon, outrage turned into action. A remarkably diverse set of organizations and constituencies began to mobilize advocacy campaigns just days after the Zero Tolerance policy was made public.[36] Even Trump loyalists began to quietly distance themselves from the policy and counseled the White House to retract or substantially revise the family separation strategy.[37] Soon, hostility to the policy reached a crescendo and after just 6 weeks after the Zero Tolerance policy was implemented border-wide, President Trump ordered that the policy be terminated.[38]

The precise number of children separated from their parents or legal guardians remains elusive but estimates have fun between 3,000 and 7,000.[39] This was due in part to multiple failures in maintaining the record of which child belonged to which parent or guardian. After more than 5 years, there remain several hundred children who have not yet been reunited with their families.[40]

Distinguishing Humanitarian Concerns from Immigration Policy

The mistreatment of children should never again be used as an instrument of immigration policy. The Zero Tolerance experience made that clear. However, there are other aspects of this experience that may also hold important lessons for the advocacy community. In particular, the response to the family separations was instructive in how to mobilize humanitarian impulses in ways that transcend political ideology and in turn, facilitate collective action involving diverse political constituencies.

Advocates opposing the Zero Tolerance policy were largely successful in making a sharp distinction between humanitarian considerations and immigration policy per se. There was a clear emphasis on the treatment of children and not the divisive politics of immigration control. The humanitarian arguments supporting improved custodial conditions for migrant children in general and the termination of the Zero Tolerance policy in particular were based on two humanitarian themes. First, there was an explicit focus on the acute and prolonged psychological damage done to children by forcibly separating them from their parents.[41] Medical groups, including the American Academy of Pediatrics, called on a broad, technical literature to support this argument.[42–44] Second, advocates, including religious organizations, recognized that beyond technical damage concerns, the widespread separation of families on the border violated deeply held moral values.[45,46] The cruelty inherent in forcibly separating a child from their parent was repulsive to wide swaths of the American public.[47,48] This response continued to gain force as images and audio of sobbing children began to trickle and then stream from the border.[49] These two humanitarian strategies have also been extended further[50] and continue to prove useful in elevating the custodial needs of migrant children in detention. However, this disassociation of humanitarian issues and immigration policy, albeit useful in the Zero Tolerance case, should be considered carefully as it can create tensions with progressive advocacy positions that expressly rely on humanitarian considerations to advance immigration policy reform.

Addressing the Responsibility of Parents

Advocacy for unaccompanied migrant children is commonly greeted by the concern that parents of these children bear the primary responsibility for the predicament the children face in border detention.[51] This, in turn, can easily translate into a subtle but consequential disavowal of US government responsibility for the care of detained children. The challenge for advocacy is in acknowledging that the parents may, at some basic level, be *responsible* for their child's predicament, but that this does not mean that they were *irresponsible* in permitting their child's unaccompanied entry into the United States and detention. The question of irresponsibility pivots on the reasons why families have resorted to unaccompanied child migration, reasons too often based on fleeing extreme poverty and violence.[52,53] These motivations coupled with US immigration policies that make it easier to be released into the United States as an unaccompanied child than as a family have created strong incentives for unaccompanied child migration. In this manner, unaccompanied child migration far more commonly reflects parental desperation than neglect, a reality that can make child migration, with all its heartbreaking character, a deeply responsible parental act.

Child Agency and Resilience

There is also a tension that can arise when advocates portray UCs solely as passive victims.[54] While appealing at times, this advocacy posture can discount children's intrinsic agency and ignore the reality that many UCs, particularly older adolescents, have participated centrally in the myriad decisions that have shaped their journey to the United States.[55–57] In addition, older UCs reveal remarkable resilience and commonly understand that being apprehended and held in a BP facility is the first procedural step in their quest for release to relatives or sponsors in the United States.[58] Although these considerations do not in any way diminish UC claims to just and humane treatment, they do underscore the need for advocates to appreciate the complex interaction between capability and vulnerability[59] that defines the challenge of caring for UCs in detention.

ADVOCACY OPPORTUNITIES FOR REFORM
The Flores Settlement Agreement

In 1985, Jenny Flores, a 15-year-old girl fleeing a violent civil war in El Salvador was arrested and detained for 2 months in substandard conditions by the Immigration and Naturalization Service, a precursor agency to the Department of Homeland Security. Her case laid the basis for what became a class action lawsuit on behalf of migrant children detained by the US government. After a decade of litigation, a settlement was reached in Federal Court, known as the Flores Settlement Agreement (FSA),[60] which outlined for the first time the basic principles and custodial standards for migrant children in detention.[61]

The federal courts have continued to serve as the most important guarantor of humane treatment for children in immigration detention. The FSA has provided a foundation for a series of subsequent court rulings that have continued to improve the standards of care and the procedures and the timeliness of release, for both UCs and families.[62] It has also served as a basis for ongoing mediation efforts between the government and advocates to address alleged violations and the need to further improve custodial conditions.[25] As a result, the FSA remains an essential tool for the continuing improvement of custodial care for UCs in detention.

Border Patrol Custodial Care

There is a humanitarian imperative to continually improve the custodial conditions of UCs in BP detention. This entails a commitment to fully implement the standards of care mandated by the FSA. However, the FSA represents the minimum standard of humanitarian provision, not the optimal. Accordingly, efforts to continually improve custodial conditions remain essential, particularly in mitigating the mental health implications of traumatic migratory experiences and detention.

Overcrowding

Of special concern is the prevention of overcrowding, the one condition that can unravel virtually all custodial systems. This implies an ability to quickly flex not only housing capabilities but also hygiene, sanitation, nutrition, and medical services, in response to increased flows of UCs. Since 2014, CBP and ORR have had a mixed record of responding to rapid increases in UC and family apprehensions.[63–65] These agencies will require greater resources and operational flexibility to plan for and deploy expanded custodial capabilities.

Caregivers

As long as children are being held in CBP custody, there must be a commitment to staff the relevant facilities with dedicated childcare workers, or caregivers, who are responsible for providing direct humanitarian services to the children.[25] Although working under CBP supervision and security, the caregivers represent a more appropriate workforce for childcare than CBP agents or contracted guard services. Moreover, caregivers represent virtually the only means by which CBP could integrate services that attend more fully to the mental health of UCs. These could include specialized child-friendly physical and procedural enhancements as well as a full range of pragmatic, trauma-informed care strategies, including entry orientation, recreational or creative activities, and the identification of distressed children in need of urgent mental health intervention.

Office of Refugee Resettlement

As the federal entity charged with the prolonged care and reunification of UCs in US detention, ORR must have sufficient custodial capacity to provide appropriate services for whatever number of UCs are apprehended at the border. ORRs establishment of the EISs was an effective emergency response to a dramatic increase in ORR holding and processing capacities in early 2021. Although efforts to enhance services at the EISs and ICFs are beneficial, the custodial standards do not meet the housing and custodial standards that ORR has long set for its licensed custodial programs.[66–68] There is a danger, therefore, that the EISs, rather than being considered a temporary, emergency response, are maintained as a sustained alternative to licensed facilities. The EISs, therefore, should be replaced by full-service, licensed facilities.

Whole Government Reforms

Beyond improving conditions in current CBP and ORR care, it is essential that broader systemic reforms be actively explored. These systemic initiatives must involve multiple federal agencies, an approach often labeled "whole government" reforms. In large measure, the current detention structures for migrants were created as a law enforcement system designed primarily to hold and process adult

Mexican men looking for work in the United States. The major demographic shift toward UCs and families since 2014 has placed an unprecedented burden on CBP to house, process, and provide appropriate care for hundreds of thousands of children each year.

Alternative structures should be explored,[69] particularly those that would reduce or eliminate CBP custody of UCs. For example, procedures could be revised so that ORR could assume custody of UCs directly from the field. CBP would still be required to conduct apprehensions and facilitate immediate medical referral for any child with an acute medical need. However, unlike the current system, UCs could then be taken for initial intake and all custodial care to an ORR facility, largely bypassing CBP custodial requirements. This type of structural reform would require a whole government approach with coordinated revisions in processing and custodial responsibilities across multiple agencies. While difficult at times, this type of structural reform would not only allow CBP to focus more directly on its primary security role but would also hold the greatest promise of substantially improving the custodial conditions for UCs coming into US detention.

Separation from Trusted Adults

A child who has been apprehended while in the care of a grandmother, adult sibling, or any other trusted adult that is not a parent or legal guardian will be routinely separated from the trusted adult, newly considered an unaccompanied child, and transferred to ORR care. Often, the trusted adult has been the primary caretaker of the child in the home country. This practice is due to the current interpretation of the Trafficking Victims Protection Reauthorization Act of 2008 which created procedures for processing UCs in response to their vulnerability to trafficking and other forms of exploitation.[70] However, greater efforts could be made to revise these procedures in ways that would, for selected cases, permit the child and trusted adult to be considered a family unit and not separated at the border. This would require BP and ORR to coordinate vetting procedures to identify quickly, but fully, the identity of the trusted adult and their relationship to the child. Not only would these revised procedures reduce the number of UCs requiring ORR care but they would also prove less psychologically damaging to the child.

SUMMARY

In many ways, supportive advocacy for migrant children has had to confront the collision of two disparate themes in public life. There is the idealized American vision of the child, an image imbued with the innocence, the beauty, the promise of childhood.[71–73] Then, there is the American image of the southern migrant, an image that has been battered by highly divisive political rhetoric grounded in the special kind of resentment reserved for the intruder, the outsider, the other.[74] The tension between these two perspectives has generated both a variety of humanitarian inadequacies and opportunities for continued remedial action. In addition, there are substantial opportunities to improve care through whole government reforms that better coordinate the procedures and custodial practices used by the relevant federal agencies.

However, in the end, the greatest challenge for advocacy will be to navigate an alpine policy landscape defined by a divisive politics, the complex technical requirements of caring for children, and a public struggling to find some acceptable expression of humanitarian compassion for children seeking a new life in the United States, on their own.

CLINICS CARE POINTS

- Clinicians caring form migrant children should inquire whether they were held in government custody and are in need of legal or social services.
- Unaccompanied children may be held in shelters far from the border and present for care without parental presence.
- Clinicians should familiarize themselves with their state policies for financing medical services for migrant children.

DISCLOSURE

The author has nothing to disclose.

REFERENCES

1. Okrent D. The Guarded Gate: Bigotry, Eugenics, and the Law That Kept Two Generations of Jews, Italians, and Other European Immigrants out of America. Scribner 2019.
2. Linton JM, Nagda J, Falusi OO. Advocating for Immigration Policies that Promote Children's Health. Pediatr Clin North Am 2019;66(3):619–40.
3. Linton JM, Griffin M, Shapiro AJ. Detention of Immigrant Children. Pediatrics 2017;139(5):e20170483.
4. Linton JM, Kennedy E, Shapiro A, et al. Unaccompanied children seeking safe haven: Providing care and supporting well-being of a vulnerable population. Child Youth Serv Rev 2018;122–32. https://doi.org/10.1016/j.childyouth.2018.03.043.
5. Kandel WA. Unaccompanied alien children: an overview.; 2021:1-42. Available at: https://crsreports.congress.gov. Accessed July 13, 2022.
6. U.S. Border Patrol Southwest Border Apprehensions by Sector | U.S. Customs and Border Protection. Available at: https://www.cbp.gov/newsroom/stats/southwest-land- border-encounters/usbp-sw-border-apprehensions. Accessed July 13, 2022.
7. Southwest Land Border Encounters (By Component) | U.S. Customs and Border Protection. Available at: https://www.cbp.gov/newsroom/stats/southwest-land-border- encounters-by-component. Accessed July 13, 2022.
8. Erdal MB, Oeppen C. Forced to leave? The discursive and analytical significance of describing migration as forced and voluntary. J Ethn Migr Stud 2018;44(6):981–98.
9. Rodriguez N, Urrutia-Rojas X, Gonzalez LR. Unaccompanied minors from the Northern Central American countries in the migrant stream: social differentials and institutional contexts. J Ethn Migr Stud 2019;45(2):218–34.
10. World Bank. Poverty Headcount Ratio at National Poverty Lines. Available at: https://data.worldbank.org/indicator/SI.POV.NAHC?end=2020&start=2020&view=map&yea r_high_desc=true. Accessed July 14, 2022.
11. Munoz E. The geography of intergenerational mobility in Latin America and the caribbean. World Bank Group. Policy Research Working Paper 10036. 2022.
12. UNICEF. On my mind: promoting, protecting and caring for children's mental health. UNICEF; 2021. Available at: https://www.unicef.org/reports/state-worldschildren-2021. Accessed July 13, 2022.

13. Pons D. Climate Extremes, Food Insecurity, and Migration in Central America: A Complicated Nexus. migrationpolicy.org. Available at: https://www. migrationpolicy.org/article/climate-food-insecurity-migration-central-   america-guatemala. Accessed July 14, 2022.

14. Evoy CM, Hideg G. Global violent deaths 2017: time to decide. small arms survey; 2017. Available at: https://www.smallarmssurvey.org/resource/global-violent-deaths-2017.

15. Bank W. Worldwide Governance Indicators. Available at: http://info.worldbank. org/governance/wgi/index.aspx#home   http://data.worldbank.org/data-catalog/worldwide-governance-indicators. Accessed May 4, 2015.

16. Characteristics of Separated Children in ORR's Care: June 27, 2018–November 15. 2020. Available at: https://oig.hhs.gov/oei/reports/OEI-BL-20-00680.asp. Accessed July 15, 2022.

17. Campana P. Human smuggling: Structure and mechanisms. Crime Justice 2020; 49(1):471–519.

18. Greenfield V, Nunez-Neto B, Mitch I, et al. Human smuggling and associated revenues: what do or can we know about routes from Central America to the United States? RAND Corporation; 2019. Available at. https://doi.org/10.7249/RR2852. Accessed July 13, 2022.

19. Chang KSG, Tsang S, Chisolm-Straker M. Child trafficking and exploitation: Historical roots, preventive policies, and the Pediatrician's role. Curr Probl Pediatr Adolesc Health Care 2022;52(3):101167.

20. Haddal CC. Border security: the role of the U.S. Border Patrol. :41.

21. Marquez-Avila M. No More Hieleras: Doe v. Kelly's Fight for Constitutional Rights at the Border. UCLA L Rev 2019;66:818–59.

22. Directive 2210-004-CBP Enhanced Medical Efforts. U.S. Customs and Border Protection, Department of Homeland Security. 2020. Available at: https://www. cbp.gov/document/directives/directive-2210-004-cbp-enhanced-medical-efforts. Accessed July 14, 2022.

23. Office of Inspector General Department of Homeland Security. Rio Grande Valley Area Border Patrol Struggles with High Volumes of Detainees and Cases of Prolonged Detention but Has Taken Consistent Measures to Improve Conditions in Facilities. 2022. Available at: https://www.oig.dhs.gov. Accessed July 14, 2022.

24. Americans for Immigrant Justice. Do My Rights Matter? The mistreatment of unaccompanied children in CBP custody. 2020. Available at: https://aijustice.org/do-my-rights-matter-the-mistreatment-of-unaccompanied-children-in-cbp-custody/. Accessed July 14, 2022.

25. CBP Settlement Agreement Flores v. Garland, Case No. 2:85-cv-4544 (C.D. Cal.). Available at: https://www.aila.org/infonet/flores-   v-reno-settlement-agreement. Accessed July 14, 2022.

26. Children Entering the United States Unaccompanied. Available at: https://www. acf.hhs.gov/orr/policy-guidance/children-entering-united-states-unaccompanied. Accessed July 14, 2022.

27. Greenberg M. U.S. Government Makes Significant Strides in Receiving Unaccompanied Children but Major Challenges Remain. Available at: https://www. migrationpolicy.org/news/unaccompanied-children-   emergency-intake-site-challenges. Accessed July 14, 2022.

28. Emergency Intake Sites for Unaccompanied Children. KIND. Available at: https:// supportkind.org/resources/emergency-intake-sites-for-unaccompanied-children/. Accessed July 14, 2022.

29. Office of Refugee Resettlement, Administration for Childrn and Families. ORR Field guidance #13, Emergency Intake Sites (EIS) Instructions and Standards. Published online April 30, 2021.

30. Women's Refugee Commission; First Focus on Children. Unaccompanied children in emergency intake site (EIS) facilities-A progress report.; 2022.

31. Kandel WA. The Trump Administration's "Zero Tolerance" Immigration Enforcement Policy. Rep Congr Res Serv R 2018;1–24. Published online.

32. Jacob S. Separated: Inside an American Tragedy.

33. Qiu L. Republicans Misplace Blame for Splitting Families at the Border. The New York Times. Available at: https://www.nytimes.com/2018/06/14/us/politics/fact-check-republicans-family- separations-border.html. Accessed July 14, 2022.

34. Shear MD, Benner K, Schmidt MS. 'We Need to Take Away Children,' No Matter How Young, Justice Dept. Officials Said. The New York Times. Available at: https://www.nytimes.com/2020/10/06/us/politics/family-separation-border-immigration-jeff- sessions-rod-rosenstein.html. Accessed July 14, 2022.

35. Kirstjen Nielsen Continues to Insist That There Is No Family Separation Policy. American Civil Liberties Union. Available at: https://www.aclu.org/blog/immigrants-rights/ice-and-border-patrol-abuses/kirstjen-nielsen-   continues-insist-there-no. Accessed July 14, 2022.

36. Angered by family separations at the border, advocacy groups plan White House protest June 30 - The Washington Post. Available at: https://www.washingtonpost.com/news/local/wp/2018/06/19/angered-by-family-separations-   at-the-border-advocacy-groups-plan-white-house-protest-june-30/. Accessed July 14, 2022.

37. Shear MD, Stolberg SG, Kaplan T. G.O.P. Moves to End Trump's Family Separation Policy, but Can't Agree How. The New York Times. Available at: https://www.nytimes.com/2018/06/19/us/politics/trump-immigration-children-separated-families.html. Accessed July 14, 2022.

38. Trump signs order ending his policy of separating families at the border, but reprieve may be temporary. Washington Post. Available at: https://www.washingtonpost.com/politics/trump-signs-   order-ending-his-policy-of-separating-families-at-the-border-but-reprieve-may-be-   temporary/2018/06/20/663025ae-74a0-11e8-b4b7-308400242c2e_story.html. Accessed July 14, 2022.

39. Separated Children Placed in Office of Refugee Resettlement Care (OEIBL-18-00511; 01/19). Available at: https://oig.hhs.gov/oei/reports/oei-BL-18-00511.asp. Accessed July 15, 2022.

40. Interagency task force on the reunification of families. Interim Progress Report.; 2021. Available at: https://www.dhs.gov/sites/default/files/publications/21_0826_s1_interim-progress-report-family-reunification-task-force.pdf. Accessed July 13, 2022.

41. Monico C, Rotabi K, Vissing Y, et al. Forced Child-Family Separations in the Southwestern US Border Under the "Zero-Tolerance" Policy: the Adverse Impact on Well- Being of Migrant Children (Part 2). J Hum Rights Soc Work 2019;4(3):180–91.

42. Kraft C. AAP Statement Opposing Separation of Children and Parents at the Border. Available at: https://www.aap.org/en/news-room/news-releases/aap/2018/aapstatement-opposing-separation-of-children-and-parents-at-the-border/. Accessed July 13, 2022.

43. Cohodes EM, Kribakaran S, Odriozola P, et al. Migration-related trauma and mental health among migrant children emigrating from Mexico and Central America to the United States: Effects on developmental neurobiology and implications for policy. Dev Psychobiol 2021;63(6):e22158.

44. Menjívar C, Perreira KM. Undocumented and unaccompanied: children of migration in the European Union and the United States. J Ethn Migr Stud 2019;45(2): 197–217.

45. US bishops condemn immigration policies that separate families at border. National Catholic Reporter. Available at: https://www.ncronline.org/news/people/us-bishops-condemn-immigration-policies-separate- families-border. Accessed July 15, 2022.

46. Evangelical Leaders Urge President Trump To Keep Families Together. Evangelical Immigration Table. Available at: https://evangelicalimmigrationtable.com/evangelical-leaders-urge-president-trump-to-keep- families-together/. Accessed July 15, 2022.

47. Laura Bush. Separating children from their parents at the border 'breaks my heart.' Washington Post. Available at: https://www.washingtonpost.com/opinions/laura-bush-separating-children-   from-their-parents-at-the-border-breaks-my-heart/2018/06/17/f2df517a-7287-11e8-9780-   b1dd6a09b549_story.html. Accessed July 14, 2022.

48. Catholic bishops across U.S. condemn separation of migrant children. America Magazine. Available at: https://www.americamagazine.org/politics-society/2018/06/18/catholic-bishops-across-us- condemn-separation-migrant-children. Accessed July 14, 2022.

49. Kelly ML. Migrant Children Heard Crying On Tape Are The Voices "Left Out" Of Conversation. NPR. Available at: https://www.npr.org/2018/06/19/621579091/migrant-children-heard- crying-on-tape-are-the-voices-left-out-conversation. Accessed July 14, 2022.

50. Oberg C, Kivlahan C, Mishori R, et al. Treatment of Migrant Children on the US Southern Border Is Consistent With Torture. Pediatrics 2021;147(1). e2020012930.

51. Secretary Kirstjen M. Nielsen Statement on Passing of Eight Year Old Guatemalan Child| Homeland Security. Available at: https://www.dhs.gov/news/2018/12/26/secretary-kirstjen-m-nielsen-statement-passing-eight-   year-old-guatemalan-child. Accessed July 14, 2022.

52. How To Argue Asylum Seekers Aren't "Irresponsible" For Bringing Kids To The US. Bustle. Available at: https://www.bustle.com/p/how-to-argue-asylum-seekers- arent-irresponsible-for-bringing-kids-to-the-us-15913325. Accessed July 14, 2022.

53. Stinchcomb D, Hershberg E. Unaccompanied Migrant Children from Central America: Context, Causes, and Responses. SSRN Electron J 2014. https://doi.org/10.2139/ssrn.2524001.

54. O'Connell Davidson J. Moving children? Child trafficking, child migration, and child rights. Crit Soc Policy 2011;31(3):454–77.

55. Thompson A, Torres RM, Swanson K, et al. Re-conceptualising agency in migrant children from Central America and Mexico. J Ethn Migr Stud 2019;45(2):235–52.

56. Terrio S, Somers A, Faries O, Menjivar C, Krause EL, Lustig S. Voice, Agency and Vulnerability: the Immigration of Children through Systems of Protection and Enforcement. Int Migr 2010;49:1–23.

57. Uehling GL. The International Smuggling of Children: Coyotes, Snakeheads, and the Politics of Compassion. Anthropol Q 2008;81(4):833–71.

58. Browne DT, Smith JA, Basabose JDD. Refugee Children and Families during the COVID-19 Crisis: A Resilience Framework for Mental Health. J Refug Stud 2021; 34(1):1138–49.

59. Christensen PH. Childhood and the Cultural Constitution of Vulnerable Bodies. In: Prout A, Campling J, editors. The body, childhood and society. Palgrave Macmillan UK; 2000. p. 38–59. https://doi.org/10.1007/978-0-333-98363-8_3. Accessed July 13, 2022.
60. Peck SH, Harrington B. The "Flores Settlement" and Alien Families Apprehended at the U.S. Border: Frequently Asked Questions. cong Res Serv. Available at: https://www.everycrsreport.com/reports/R45297.html. Accessed July 15, 2022.
61. López RM. Codifying the Flores Settlement Agreement : Seeking to Protect Immigrant Children in U . S . Custody. Marquette L Rev 2012;95(4):1635–77.
62. Schrag PG. Baby jails: the fight to end the incarceration of refugee children in America. University of California Press; 2020.
63. Sullivan E, Kanno-Youngs Z, Broadwater L. Overcrowded Border Jails Give Way to Packed Migrant Child Shelters. The New York Times. Available at: https://www.nytimes.com/2021/05/07/us/politics/migrant-children-shelters.html. Published May 7, 2021. Accessed July 14, 2022.
64. Lind D. "No Good Choices": HHS Is Cutting Safety Corners to Move Migrant Kids Out of Overcrowded Facilities. ProPublica. Available at: https://www.propublica.org/article/no-good-choices-hhs-is-cutting-safety-corners-to-move-migrant-kids-out-of-overcrowded-facilities. Accessed July 14, 2022.
65. Kelly JV. Management alert - DHS needs to address dangerous overcrowding among single adults at El Paso Del norte (redacted). 2019; Available at: https://www.oig.dhs.gov/sites/default/files/assets/Mga/2019/oig-19-46-may19-mgmtalert.pdf. Accessed July 13, 2022.
66. Allain M. Government Accountability Project Raises Ongoing Concerns about Treatment of Unaccompanied Immigrant Children at HHS Emergency Intake Sites. Government Accountability Project. Available at: https://whistleblower.org/press-release/press-release-government-accountability-project-raises-ongoing-concerns-about-treatment-of-unaccompanied-immigrant-children-at-hhs-emergency-intake-sites/. Accessed July 14, 2022.
67. Never Again: Emergency Intake Sites (EISs) Harm Immigrant Children. National Center for Youth Law. Available at: https://youthlaw.org/news/never-again-emergency-intake-sites-eiss-harm-immigrant-children. Accessed July 14, 2022.
68. Class-Action Suit Strengthens Protections For Immigrant Children. National Center for Youth Law. Available at: https://youthlaw.org/news/class-action-suit-strengthens-protections-immigrant-children. Accessed July 14, 2022.
69. International Detention Coalition. Gaining Ground: Promising Practice to Reduce and End Immigration Detention. 2022. Available at: https://idcoalition.org/publication/gaining-ground-promising-practice-to-reduce-end-immigration-detention/. Accessed July 14, 2022.
70. Estin AL. Child migrants and child welfare: toward a best interests approach. Wash U Glob Stud Rev 2018;17(3):589–614.
71. Zelizer VA. Pricing the priceless child: the changing social value of children. Princeton, NJ: Princeton University Press; 1994.
72. Gordon Linda. The Perils of Innocence, or What's Wrong with Putting Children First. J Hist Child Youth 2008;1(3):331–50.
73. Wise PH. Child Beauty, Child Rights, and the Devaluation of Women. Health Hum Serv News. 1(4):472-476.
74. Finley L, Esposito L. The Immigrant as Bogeyman: Examining Donald Trump and the Right's Anti-immigrant, Anti-PC Rhetoric. Humanity Soc 2020;44(2):178–97.

Global Child Advocacy

Advocacy for Global Tobacco Control and Child Health

Felicia Scott-Wellington, MD, Elissa A. Resnick, MPH, Jonathan D. Klein, MD, MPH*

KEYWORDS

- Tobacco control • Global tobacco advocacy • Adolescent health • Addiction

KEY POINTS

- Tobacco and secondhand smoke remain leading causes of death and illnesses including cancer, asthma exacerbations, chronic bronchitis, and increased risks of heart disease and stroke.
- The tobacco industry has historically targeted vulnerable populations including children and adolescents with deceptive advertising, misleading claims, and promotional campaigns.
- Electronic cigarettes have become more popular due to the tobacco industry's portrayal of these products as "safer" despite increasing evidence that these products pose serious health risks.
- While regulations have been somewhat successful in protecting youths from combustible cigarettes, they have been slow to update to protect youths from newer products including electronic cigarettes.
- Preventing tobacco use and addiction to nicotine is key to protect health. Advocates must remain persistent in their efforts to counter industry tactics and protect public health.

HISTORY OF TOBACCO

Nicotana is a genus of annual and perennial plants that encompass over 60 species, known as tobacco plants. Tobacco plants are native to the Americas, and the cultivation of tobacco can be traced back several thousand years BC.[1] Around 1 BC Mayans in Central America began smoking tobacco leaves during sacred and religious ceremonies.[2] Tribal healers also found tobacco plants helpful for various illnesses, including asthma, ear pain, bowel problems, toothaches, headaches, and burns.[2]

After spreading throughout the Americas, in the late 15th century European explorers brought tobacco leaves and seeds back to Europe. Tobacco did not gain popularity in Europe until Jean Nicot, from whom its name is derived, presented the plant to the queen of France, who endorsed the plant for its healing powers. It was

Department of Pediatrics, University of Illinois at Chicago, 1206 CSB MC 856 840 S. Wood Street, Chicago, IL 60612, USA
* Corresponding author.
E-mail address: jonklein@uic.edu

Pediatr Clin N Am 70 (2023) 117–135
https://doi.org/10.1016/j.pcl.2022.09.011
0031-3955/23/© 2022 Elsevier Inc. All rights reserved.

viewed as a panacea for all disease and pain, and quickly spread throughout Europe, Asia, and the rest of the world.[3] In the United States, tobacco use through most of the 19th century was limited to chewing tobacco. In 1881, the invention of the automatic cigarette rolling machine accelerated a shift to cigarettes. In the early 20th century, public health efforts to stop the spread of influenza and tuberculosis by discouraging spittoon use furthered the use of combustible tobacco.[4]

TOBACCO INDUSTRY APPEALS TO CONSUMERS

Throughout modern history, tobacco companies have appealed to consumers in ways that undermine public health efforts. In the early 1900s, after advocates successfully banned cigarettes in 15 states,[5] tobacco companies argued that cigarette bans were unpatriotic in the face of World War I. When postwar data showed a connection between smoking and poor health,[6,7] tobacco companies responded by using physicians' endorsements and false health claims in their advertisements.[8,9]

Starting with Hollywood's "Golden Age" (1920s–1960s), tobacco companies partnered with movie studios to portray smoking as glamorous.[10] Actors were instructed to smoke on screen and to appear in tobacco ads in exchange for funding for the studios. At the same time, the industry continued to characterize tobacco as patriotic through World War II. Cigarette rations, established by Congress during WWI, were increased for soldiers during WWII.[11]

Smoking rates peaked in the 1960s, just before the first Surgeon General's report, with more than 40% of adults smoking cigarettes.[12] By appealing to consumers' patriotism, glamor, and even health, tobacco companies have continually stayed steps ahead of public health and regulatory efforts to decrease smoking.

RECOGNITION OF INDUSTRY AS BAD ACTORS

In the early 1950s, additional evidence showing a connection between smoking and cancer was emerging. The tobacco industry responded by forming the Tobacco Industry Research Committee in 1953, an organization dedicated to attacking scientific studies.[13] The companies created and promoted filtered cigarettes as "healthy," even though internal industry documents revealed that tobacco companies knew that those who smoked filtered cigarettes inhaled as much or more tar, nicotine, and other toxins as those who smoked unfiltered cigarettes, and that adding filters did not make cigarettes safer.[14]

In 1958, the tobacco industry formed the Tobacco Institute, which supported the Tobacco Industry Research Committee's attempts to undermine public health. The Tobacco Institute claimed that antitobacco advocates and scientists were distorting their findings. In a key strategy to what has become known as the "Tobacco Playbook," they argued that proposed tobacco control measures were supported by inconclusive evidence; creating an artificial "conflict" over the science, and successfully delaying or avoiding effective regulation. In addition to discrediting scientists, the Tobacco Institute framed smoking as a personal choice rather than an addiction, and they argued that health problems afflicting smokers were due to heredity and other lifestyle choices.[15]

Despite this, public health efforts made progress in the latter half of the 20th century. Key events included the:

- 1964 report "Smoking and Health: Report of the Advisory Committee of the Surgeon General of the Public Health Service,"
- 1965 Federal Cigarette Labeling and Advertising Act,

- 1969 Public Health Cigarette Smoking Act
- 1971 ban on television cigarette advertisements,
- 1975 removal of cigarettes from armed forces troop rations
- 1998 Tobacco Master Settlement Agreement
- 2005 World Health Organization Framework Convention on Tobacco Control (FCTC) and Tobacco Free Initiative launched

In response to many of these milestone events, the industry remained nimble. Movie and television product placement replaced traditional advertisements, allowing tobacco companies to continue to promote their products. Though removed from official rations, free cigarettes and tobacco-branded materials were sent to deployed troops,[11] and cigarette branded "Welcome Home" events were sponsored on US military bases for returning troops.[16] Similar exploitation of loopholes in public health efforts to protect young people from tobacco and nicotine persist today, with the industry heavily modifying and marketing products that escaped regulations, pivoting to new products, encouraging "debate" over products' harms and benefits, and marketing to youth.

NEW PRODUCTS

As regulation was aimed at limiting marketing of traditional combustible tobacco products to children, the industry developed alternative approaches to take advantage of regulatory loopholes. For example, as flavorings were eliminated from cigarettes, tobacco companies added flavorings known to be attractive to youth to alternative products, including snuff pouches, chewing tobacco, and little cigars (which are relatively indistinguishable from cigarettes.)[17]

In the past decade, these strategies have also led to the rapid spread of electronic cigarettes/vaping products. Clever and well-funded social media campaigns market these products to youths.[18] E-cigarettes are available in a range of appealing flavors. As a result of misleading marketing, nearly 40% of youths believe that using e-cigarettes are not harmful.[19] Additionally, e-cigarette products have not been subject to the same regulatory scrutiny as traditional cigarettes. Some tobacco control advocates have promoted the potential for e-cigarettes as harm reduction options or as cessation aids for addicted smokers. However, evidence has mounted for their negative health effects and has shown that they consistently prevent quitting, rather than facilitating cessation.[20] Notwithstanding this evidence, the industry has co-opted harm reduction framing of e-cigarettes, delayed effective regulatory action, and vigorously promoted and marketed e-cigarettes to youth, using fruit and candy flavors and creative packaging. As has been the case throughout the history of tobacco control, the promotion of "scientific controversy" has delayed attempts to limit e-cigarette availability and accessibility, allowing the industry to prey on and addict young consumers.[21]

Tobacco as a Global Issue: Geographic Variation

Tobacco use is ubiquitous, with an estimated 1.3 billion tobacco users worldwide. Geographic and cultural variation exist: South-East Asia is one of the largest tobacco epidemic regions, as both a producer and consumer of tobacco.[22] In 2000, the South-East Asia region had tobacco use rates nearing 50%, the highest of any WHO region.[23] Although these rates declined in recent decades thanks to vigorous tobacco control efforts (see case study 1 for pediatric's contributions to this advocacy) approximately 25% of adults aged 15 and older and one-third of children ages 13–15 report using tobacco.[23] Despite these declining trends, smokeless tobacco promotion is growing in South East Asia, and 81% of smokeless user live in this region.[24]

In Europe, tobacco use prevalence in both genders is high, with rates nearing 30% in men and 20% in women. A slow decline in tobacco use among European women leaves them with usage rates substantially higher than any other WHO region.[25] Tobacco use in Europe was once largely a male-dominated phenomenon; however, the gap between genders is now very small in many countries.[26] In Sweden and Norway, the prevalence of daily smoking is higher in women than in men, highlighting the need to explore gender targeted regional interventions. Tobacco use among adolescents in Europe is rising, with countries such as Lithuania, Latvia, and Czech Republic having adolescent use rates mirroring that of adults.[27]

The WHO AFRO region has one of the lowest smoking prevalence regions worldwide. However, the number of tobacco users in both the AFRO and the Middle East and North Africa (MENA) regions continues to steadily rise; these are the only 2 regions that have not seen an overall decline in smoking prevalence rates. The AFRO region's booming adolescent population makes it a targeted area for tobacco industry efforts. Inconsistent regulations, low cost, and lack of enforcement create a perfect storm, acting as a driver for increasing youth usage and addiction in these areas.[28,29]

The Americas Region has shown the most dramatic decline in tobacco prevalence, with tobacco use rates dropping to 21% in 2010 and 16% in 2020.[30] Despite these declining numbers, 34 million US adults smoke, 50 million US nonsmokers are exposed to secondhand smoke, and there are more than 70 million smokers in Latin America.[31] Throughout the region men have higher rates than women, but rates in Latin America and the Caribbean closely follow Europe's trend, with women's rates second highest among all regions. There are high rates of youth initiation in the US and the rest of the Americas with Jamaica, Colombia, and Chile having the highest rates of youth tobacco consumption (**Fig. 1**).[31]

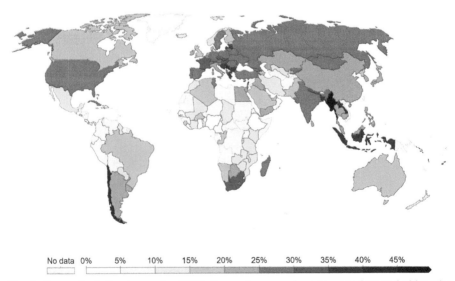

No data 0%   5%   10%   15%   20%   25%   30%   35%   40%   45%

Fig. 1. Share of adults who smoke, 2018. Share of men and women aged 15 and older who smoke any tobacco product on a daily or nondaily basis. It excludes smokeless tobacco use. (Hannah Ritchie and Max Roser (2013) - "Smoking". Published online at OurWorldInData.org. Retrieved from: 'https://ourworldindata.org/smoking' [Online Resource].)

Different Tobacco Products are Used in Different Countries and Cultures

Tobacco products use is influenced by cultural and regional differences. In the US, Latin America, the Caribbean, and Europe, factory-manufactured tobacco products such as cigarettes, cigars, and pipes still remain the most popular, however, in Europe roll-your-own cigarettes are used at high rates in some countries in the region. E−cigarette use has been rising globally, especially in both Europe and the Americas.

In Southeast Asia, tobacco use includes both smoking and smokeless tobacco. Smokeless products may be chewed, sniffed, or dipped. Smokeless tobacco is used by over 300 million people in 70 countries worldwide.[24] In SouthEast Asia smoking and smokeless tobacco products include, hukka (or hookah/water pipe), chilam (clay pipe), cigarettes or *bidis* (dried tobacco wrapped in tendu or temburni leaves), *khaini* (tobacco with lime), *paan masala* (tobacco wrapped in betel leaf or packed in foil), *gutkha* (mixture of tobacco and molasses), and chewing tobacco mixed with areca nuts.[2]

In all areas of the world, tobacco use has been linked to lower education, socioeconomic status, and poverty, highlighting the importance of implementing country-specific tobacco policies that reach these vulnerable populations.[32]

Table/maps of variation
https://www.thelancet.com/infographics/tobacco
https://www.cdc.gov/tobacco/global/gtss/gtssdata/index.html.

HEALTH EFFECTS OF TOBACCO

Evidence for the harmful effects of tobacco has been well documented. Virtually no level of tobacco consumption or exposure is safe. Tobacco accounts for approximately 8 million deaths worldwide per year, with more than 1 million of these from non-smokers' exposure to secondhand smoke.[33]

Nicotine is a highly addictive chemical and is both toxic and carcinogenic. Nicotine is found in all tobacco products, Its absorption through mucosal surfaces differs with product composition and PH.[34] The South-East Asian practice of adding lime or areca nuts to tobacco increases the absorption of nicotine.[34] Menthol, commonly added to many forms of tobacco, both accelerates absorption and anesthetizes and masks the harshness of tobacco products, contributing to youth addiction. Nicotine has a rapid onset of its effects, increasing adrenaline and activating dopaminergic pathways in the brain reward center, resulting in mood elevation and cognitive changes.[35] Over time, however, repeated stimulation desensitizes inhibitory GABA receptors, resulting in the cravings and dependence seen in addicted tobacco users.[36]

Cigarette smoking is still the most common form of tobacco used in the US and worldwide. The deleterious effects of tobacco smoke can be linked to disease in almost every organ system. Although longitudinal evidence is still emerging, electronic cigarette vapor also has increasingly been found to be causally associated with adverse health effects.

Tobacco smoke causes injury to lungs and airways leading to respiratory tract damage, alveolar destruction, and altered airflow resulting in:

- COPD (Chronic Obstructive Pulmonary Disease)
  - Emphysema
  - Chronic Bronchitis
- Lung Cancer
- Asthma Exacerbation

Smoke exposure also increases the risk or and severity of respiratory infections and in infants and children, as well as in adults, reflecting both the toxic effect of direct exposure and the longer-term impact on the oropharyngeal and lung microbiome.[36]

Tobacco smoke is a major cause of cardiovascular disease leading to 1 out of every 4 cardiovascular-related deaths.[37] Changes that occur include:

- Atherosclerosis
- Narrowing of vasculature
- Thickening of the blood increases risk of:
  - Heart disease
  - Stroke
  - Other cardiovascular diseases.

The inflammatory changes from smoking or from secondhand smoke exposure increase cardiovascular events (such as heart attacks) through acute, immediate vasoconstriction on exposure; it also exacerbate metabolic syndrome, contributing to diabetes and obesity,[38] and to rheumatoid arthritis.[39]

Tobacco smoke and e-cigarette vapor also contain carcinogens that damage cellular functions directly leading to a myriad of cancers including:[40]

- Lung
- Trachea
- Mouth/oropharynx
- Esophagus
- Throat
- Blood
- Colon
- Stomach
- Liver
- Pancreas

It is estimated that over 90% of lung cancers in men and 80% in women, worldwide, are directly linked to tobacco.[41] Smoking increases the risks of acquiring infectious diseases, such as tuberculosis, and further exacerbates the vascular damage from hyperglycemia is seen in diabetes (**Fig. 2**).[42]

Originally promoted as a less harmful alternative to tobacco, smokeless tobacco products have also been shown to be highly addictive, containing nicotine and carcinogenic toxins that vary across product types. Used by over 300 million users worldwide,[43] smokeless products cause cancers, cardiovascular disease, dental disease, stillbirth, premature labor, low birthweight, and other, equally devastating negative outcomes.[24]

HARMFUL EFFECTS OF MARKETING AND PROMOTION

Strong evidence has also emerged that proves that the vector for nicotine addiction and tobacco use is the advertising and marketing conducted by the industry. The 2014 US Surgeon General's report concluded: "the tobacco epidemic was initiated and has been sustained by the aggressive strategies of the tobacco industry, which has deliberately misled the public on the risks of smoking cigarettes."[39] In 2019, over 8 billion dollars was spent in tobacco advertising and marketing in the US alone.[44] Decades of tobacco industry deception and misinformation promoting choices that are harmful to health (recently defined as "commercial determinants of health")[45] continue to addict new tobacco users. Intentional marketing targeting children and

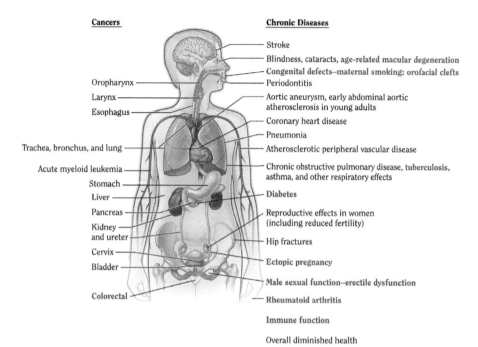

Fig. 2. The health consequences causally linked to smoking. Cancers and diseases linked to smoking. The conditions in *red* are new diseases that have been causally linked to smoking in the Surgeon General's 50th anniversary report. (*Source*: USDHHS 2004, 2006, 2012.)

adolescents has been well documented.[44,46] Vibrant colors, light devices, attractive flavors and smells, branding, and promotion of new products as harm reduction vehicles have been key to the industry's survival and profitability. New products emerge quickly with limited time for regulatory agencies to warn users or prevent their harmful effects. The tobacco industry continues to use well-calculated targeted approaches to attract unpracticed users. Celebrity influencers, scholarships, and school program sponsorship are a few tactics that directly target youth.[46] The industry's use of social media advertising platforms has been key in transforming its ability to directly attract and influence users.

Child and adolescent brains are also uniquely wired for impulsive decision making. Activation of reward pathways and slower access to frontal lobe executive functions, along with strong peer influence, makes youth particularly vulnerable to strategies designed by the industry to lure them in. Convenient single packaging, candy flavors, easy disposal, and ability to purchase products from anywhere around the world, with little to no product regulation appeals to young users, further demonstrating the industry's premeditated plan to target and influence youth.[42,46] These efforts continue to fuel the tobacco epidemic and industry success.[46]

Public Health Advocacy and Government Action are Needed

Public health advocates and researchers continuously highlight the importance of global tobacco control efforts, especially as it relates to children and adolescents. Understanding the industry's tactics of spreading misinformation and using front-groups and manufacturing "scientific" controversy to delay or avoid effective regulation is also an important and necessary part of antitobacco advocacy. Smoke-free environments increased tobacco taxation, and public health media campaigns are a few of the measures put in place to help support these efforts.[47] True antitobacco messaging under the authority of public health agencies is needed, with hard-hitting graphic testimonials that intrigue users remain the most effective messages both for prevention and tobacco cessation.[47,48]

Governmental support and funding are essential to implement effective antitobacco efforts worldwide.[33] Government actions must be unified and sustainable, collaborating with drug regulating bodies, health professional associations, nongovernmental health agencies (e.g., heart, lung, and cancer societies), and public health experts. Goals should be evidence-based and multifaceted, and include:[33]

- Maintaining youth campaign investments
- Restricting manufacturing and sales of tobacco
- Censoring or restricting tobacco marketing
- Establishing and maintaining tobacco and smoke-free facilities
- Providing addiction help and cessation support for users

Need for Advocate Support

Bans on tobacco sales and endorsement of regulatory actions that are dictated by health communities remain an uphill battle.[49] The implementation of tobacco 21 — older legal sales age — has succeeded in whole or in part in more than 40 US states, removing the legal age smokers from secondary school settings.[50] The state of California has proposed banning sales of flavored tobacco in an attempt to protect young users; however, industry push back continues to delay law implementation. An even more progressive proposal in New Zealand establishes a progressively rising age to buy cigarettes, with a goal of a lifetime tobacco ban for younger generations.[51]

Tobacco advocates must be equipped to deal with industry rebuttals as more progressive bans are replicated around the world. Relying on past experience is key, as industry tactics will be familiar, deceptive, and rooted in false arguments around freedom of choice. The industry's revolt against plain packaging further highlights this, arguing that alerting users with clear messaging is not proven to reduce tobacco use, and creates a "slippery slope" leading to universal plain packaging of all consumer products.[52] Advocates must be willing to acknowledge the potential financial impact of antitobacco restrictions on businesses, while trying to stay ahead of the industry's antics with helpful resources and solutions.[53]

INCLUDING TOBACCO CONTROL IN CARE DELIVERY AND RESEARCH

A particular opportunity for health care professional advocacy is incorporating effective tobacco control treatment and screening for secondhand smoke exposure into routine medical encounters and clinical research. Asking the right questions and delivery of effective counseling modalities has a substantial public health impact. However, despite clear evidence on the importance of limiting smoke exposure, work remains to put this into practice. Approximately 50% of children worldwide are exposed to tobacco at home.[54] Tobacco's toxins directly affect children's living environments, and these exposure increase cancer risks for both parents and children. Parental tobacco use also has been associated with children's initiation and addiction, highlighting the importance of parental tobacco screening and cessation support.[55] Despite guidelines to do so, many clinicians still do not provide evidence-based screening and counseling interventions in primary or specialty health care encounters.

Additionally, a recent review of national health policy documents of low and middle-income countries found that fewer than 10 percent of countries' newborn care guidelines addressed prenatal secondhand smoke exposure, and no guidelines addressed neonatal secondhand smoke exposure.[56] Failing to ask about smoking or secondhand smoke exposure also affects the development of new knowledge, as recently illustrated by the COVID-19 pandemic. None of the early studies about COVID-19 severity or outcomes included data about SHS exposure and few considered smoking status. The lack of SHS inclusion in surveillance made it difficult to quantify any potential relationship or to make evidence-informed recommendations about SHS exposure and COVID-19 severity risks.[57]

TOBACCO GLOBAL HEALTH ADVOCACY

Global tobacco control efforts were formalized when the World Health Organization (WHO) adopted its first treaty focused on tobacco control in 2003, The Framework Convention on Tobacco Control (FCTC).[58] The FCTC aims to lower tobacco-related mortality by regulating tobacco marketing and packaging.

WHO also established a smoke-free initiative, and identified six evidence-based country-level tobacco control measures known as MPOWER,[59] a framework for accountability to monitor the progress and effectiveness of FCTC implementation.[59] MPPOWER policies have been implemented in member countries, over 90% of whom have implemented tax and price policies, health warnings, and awareness campaigns. Two-thirds of countries have tobacco-dependence diagnosis and treatment centers and are engaged in efforts to reduce tobacco demand.[60] MPOWER's elements are (**Fig. 3**):

- *Monitor* tobacco use and prevention policies
- *Protect* people from tobacco smoke
- *Offer* to help quit tobacco use
- *Warn* about the dangers of tobacco
- *Enforce* bans on tobacco advertising, promotion, and sponsorship
- *Raise* taxes on tobacco

PEDIATRIC AND CHILD HEALTH ADVOCACY FOR TOBACCO AND SHS
Pediatrics in Action

Actionable items for children's healthcare providers include:[55]

- Inquiring about tobacco use and smoke exposure at all routine health visits
- Including tobacco prevention as routine guidance in all health visit
- Addressing caregivers tobacco dependence during health visits
- Offering tobacco dependence treatment or referral to adolescents and caregivers
- Making tobacco QUIT line referrals available
- Warning against use of electronic nicotine devices for tobacco dependence treatment
- Being ready and offering risk reduction strategies to limit tobacco smoke exposure if a commitment to smoke-free environments and cessation is not possible
- Becoming a tobacco control advocate in your community and beyond.

TOBACCO GLOBAL HEALTH ADVOCACY

- Find your tobacco-related issue

EFFECTIVE TOBACCO CONTROL MEASURES

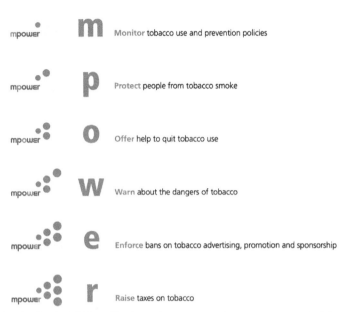

mpower **m** Monitor tobacco use and prevention policies

mpower **p** Protect people from tobacco smoke

mpower **o** Offer help to quit tobacco use

mpower **W** Warn about the dangers of tobacco

mpower **e** Enforce bans on tobacco advertising, promotion and sponsorship

mpower **r** Raise taxes on tobacco

Fig. 3. MPOWER Goals. WHO's effective tobacco control measures are prioritized by MPOWER. Image from WHO report on the global tobacco epidemic 2021: addressing new and emerging products.

Tobacco advocacy is multidimensional, advocates must, therefore, be well versed in active tobacco policy issues. The WHO MPOWER guide and the FCTC-specific objectives provide a comprehensive roadmap of issues that could be addressed. Warning against tobacco use and exposure, promoting parent and youth cessation, tackling industry misinformation, limiting marketing or access to youth, engaging awareness around tobacco's link to malnutrition, poverty, and lower SES are just a few of the key items needing advocacy in the global fight against tobacco.[61]

- Research your tobacco-related issue; know the counterarguments:

A unique aspect of tobacco control advocacy is the vigorous and well-funded protobacco voices that the industry will bring to these issues. Industry attempts to combat public health efforts are savvy. This requires child health advocates to be prepared for counter-attacks. Counter arguments are plentiful and often deny the evidence that well-studied interventions work. Industry studies, however, are often self-funded, non-peer reviewed, and flawed in the questions they ask.[52] Antitobacco advocates must keep this in mind when proposing new antitobacco initiatives. Good media skills and strong coalitions are helpful in recognizing and countering industry messaging. However, the basic steps for effective advocacy are the same as those that are needed for other child and adolescent health issues.

- Locate known antitobacco policies:

The Children's Health Insurance Plan and Reauthorization Act (CHIPRA), the Family Smoking Prevention and Tobacco Control Act, and the Affordable Care Act are a few of the US federal laws which support antitobacco efforts. The CDC Guide to Community Preventive Services provides comprehensive evidence reviews, and the American Lung Association Report Card on the annual State of Tobacco Control provides information about the implementation of policies at the State level. Globally, WHO tracks the implementation of FCTC provisions, which reflect evidence-based effective interventions to reduce the demand for tobacco. WHO's annual report on the country-level implementation of FCTC provisions provides a starting place for advocates to ensure government accountability for their commitments in selecting advocacy issues. The Bloomberg Philanthropies and their funding of the Campaign for Tobacco Free Kids and other clearinghouse groups also provides detailed information on the country adoption of policies, and potential policy stakeholders in many countries.

- Explore Coalitions; Understand stakeholders:
- Develop your ask; Make it clear:

Understanding stakeholders is essential to tobacco advocacy. When involving policy-makers or governing bodies it is important to organize data in a precise format that is easy to read and understand without extensive medical knowledge. Building a coalition and at a minimum communicating with other tobacco control stakeholders is important. Government and private sector health leaders, other professional societies, and voluntary health organizations are natural partners in mobilizing health voices against the industry's commercial interests. Develop your ask to policymakers; make it clear to elected or appointed officials what they can and should do, and why. Know the limitations of your proposal but be specific and steadfast about your ultimate goals.

- Find your legislative body:
- Contact Legislators or other key decision-makers:

Engage regional or global experts and lobby support from regulatory agencies when possible.[62] Contact with legislators or appointed government officials may offer opportunities to review current antitobacco policy and aid in the development of new initiatives. Some advocacy efforts may involve joining forces with initiatives already in place, thereby decreasing the need for repetition and extensive use of time and resources.

- Follow Up:

Tobacco companies invest billions of dollars in marketing that is purposely designed to halt public health advocacy efforts. Follow-up is, therefore, necessary to counter any industry refutation. Finding common causes with legislators and health leaders over time is possible; persistence is key, and needed, to achieve the most favorable long-term outcomes.

Tools and Resources

AAP tobacco control tool kit
https://www.tobaccofreekids.org/adhttps://www.cancer.org/vocacy-tools.

Campaign for tobacco-free kids
Campaign for Tobacco-Free Kids.
Tobacco Industry Arguments | Plain Packaging of Tobacco Products Toolkit.

Lung heart and cancer associations
American Lung Association.
   American Heart Association.
   American Cancer Society.

Action on smoking or health: American for nonsmoker rights
Action on Smoking and Health.

Case studies
1. Engaging child health and tobacco control leaders in the Asian-Pacific Region.

Evidence-based advocacy with national pediatric societies' leaders and national health ministries by the AAP Richmond Center and the Western Pacific Region WHO Tobacco-free Initiative leads to the adoption of tobacco and second-hand smoke control as a child health advocacy issue, and to the engagement of public and private collaboration between health ministries and national pediatric societies in sustainable child and family health tobacco control efforts. A small investment and the right partners can scale up child health tobacco control efforts among pediatricians world-wide, engaging stakeholders from health ministries and national pediatric societies in sustained efforts to address tobacco control in countries.

The World Health Organization regional offices can mobilize health ministries and national governments to address health priorities. The Western Pacific Regional Office (WPRO), located in Manila, in the Philippines, had strong leadership in the WHO Tobacco-free Initiative and participated in the Philippine Ambulatory Pediatric Society hosted AAP Julius B. Richmond visiting professorship by one of us (JDK) addressing children and tobacco in 2010. This led to a partnership between WPRO, the Philippine Ambulatory Pediatric Association (PAPA), the AAP Julius B. Richmond Center of Excellence, and the International Pediatric Association (IPA).

AAP, IPA, and PAPA invited national pediatric societies to identify leaders to be champions for tobacco control, and WHO-WPRO invited national government health ministries to send tobacco control staff to Protecting Children and Families from Tobacco: Leadership Training sessions which developed advocacy skills and plans for public–private partnerships to address child health and tobacco control in each country. Training focused on increasing clinicians' awareness of the impact of tobacco smoke on children and other nonsmokers, and on promoting the development of tobacco control and second-hand smoke exposure prevention curricula in schools and child health training programs. Participants from 13 countries in the region developed tobacco prevention and control advocacy plans for their national pediatric societies and other local partners/stakeholders. Half implemented plans in their countries, leading the national or subnational spread of clinical and policy champions, obtaining new national resource investments, linking to medical education institutions and national pediatric societies, and mobilizing country-specific resources and stakeholders to address tobacco and secondhand smoke in children's health care. Activities spread in more than half the countries to reach community primary care clinicians with educational interventions, and these partnerships were successful at impacting population health and health care delivery in 3 of these countries.[63]

By bringing government together with child health leaders, and helping both identify opportunities to advance tobacco control through collaborative efforts, several of the participating countries successfully launched train-the-trainers dissemination efforts, with the national champions replicating the champions' training, reaching subnational/state and local community champions and engaging effective child health advocacy voices in advancing tobacco control in their countries. Several countries received funding from their ministry of health or from private donors to support their dissemination efforts, and have remained active participants in effective tobacco prevention and control efforts for children and youth and related noncommunicable disease prevention efforts through today.

The Richmond Center was successful in similar efforts to engage pediatric society leaders in Latin America in 2012 in collaboration with the Pan American Health Organization (PAHO), and the Latin American Association of Pediatrics (ALAPE), helping 45 pediatric leaders from 12 countries develop clinical and advocacy goals for their respective countries and receive tobacco control resources to begin to actualizing these goals. Several encountered injury resistance, but were able to build effective coalitions and were prepared to counter industry efforts.

Since 2016, AAP has been supported by and partnered on champions dissemination activities with the Global Branch of the US Centers for Disease Control and Prevention (CDC) Office on Smoking and Health. CDC supports global tobacco and youth tobacco surveillance development and has worked with AAP to bring national pediatric leaders and health ministry tobacco control leaders together from more than 16 countries to support tobacco and secondhand smoke prevention programs, implement guidelines for tobacco control, and support these stakeholders' efforts to champion tobacco control in their country's health systems.[64]

1. Shedding light on the blind spots of tobacco's impact on maternal and child survival and other child health priorities.

Tobacco and second-hand smoke exposure affect child survival, nutrition, and healthy child development. US government agencies and UN agencies often minimized or avoided incorporating tobacco control messages into child survival or nutrition programmatic guidance. Advocacy with key agency staff led to reversal of USAID prohibition on tobacco control as a health and development priority, and to the recognition of tobacco-nutrition-early child development connectedness by WHO.

Early development of global health programs at the American Academy of Pediatrics (AAP) was primarily about newborn resuscitation, publications, and the iCATCH program. Starting in 2010, global programmatic growth expanded to a broader newborn survival agenda, and to immunization, tobacco control, and other noncommunicable disease efforts. As part of this growth, AAP committed staff and volunteers/members to US domestic advocacy for these global child health issues with congress and federal agencies. However, despite evidence for the harms from tobacco and secondhand smoke and AAP leadership in the USAID Survive and Thrive global development alliance, efforts to engage USAID and its in-country technical support contractors in addressing tobacco as a child survival issue were rebuffed.

In response, the American Academy of Pediatrics and the American Cancer Society Cancer Action Network organized a campaign to engage key stakeholders in helping USAID decision-makers recognize this issue as important. We identified the available evidence for the importance of tobacco control that practical steps on tobacco and secondhand smoke counseling were in the WHO Guide to *Pregnancy, Childbirth, Postpartum and Newborn* Care.[65] In contrast, efforts to prevent tobacco use and secondhand smoke (SHS) exposure were a gap in USAID's priority of ending preventable child and maternal deaths, despite USAID's call for alignment across multiple maternal and child health interventions. Not only had US government policy often encouraged tobacco agriculture and trade over health, but USAID's automated directives system (ADS) defining USAID's policies and procedures for in-country missions, was also prohibitive. Changing this became an advocacy goal.

AAP and ACS-CAN met with key USAID contractors who deliver USAID health and development investments on the ground in countries, recruiting them as allies in the health goals related to tobacco control. We also arranged constituent meetings with house and senate foreign relations appropriations committee members, held roundtable discussions, and published high-visibility blog posts calling attention to these gaps, and promoting the inclusion of evidence-based tobacco smoke exposure prevention interventions as a factor impacting prematurity, low birth weight, and other threats to maternal and child survival.[66] For example, guidelines promote breastfeeding as the best source of nutrition for infants. (WHO, UNICEF, AAP citations). Efforts to encourage breastfeeding can and should include efforts to decrease tobacco use. It was well-established that tobacco use decreases milk production.[67,68] Furthermore, while mothers who smoke are encouraged to breastfeed, toxins from cigarettes can be excreted into breast milk,[69] placing infants at risk from exposure.

A letter to USAID was developed which gained sign-on from 25 health professional organizations and several groups that partner with and support USAID's leadership in maternal and child health, encouraging the agency to use those programs to address tobacco and secondhand smoke. Over several years, these efforts were successful, with USAID agreeing to modify the ADS section on tobacco so that it both allowed and encouraged country mission directors and contractors to engage in tobacco control activities in 2016.[70] The phrase "USAID is unable to undertake a large-scale anti-tobacco effort due to staffing, programmatic, and financial constraints" was replaced by language encouraging missions to "actively implement USAID's Tobacco Policy commitment."

This change allowed national stakeholders in child survival and tobacco control to seek partnerships with USAID and its contractors in countries, and the coalition that did the advocacy work in the US also informed their networks and partner societies in other nations about USAID's availability as a tobacco control partner. AAP, in partnership with the International Pediatric Association continues to advocate for WHO, UNICEF, and other stakeholders to promote comprehensive approaches to prevention, including tobacco control, in other child survival, nutrition, and well-being programs.[71]

Lessons Learned

1. Know the evidence; and the politics—what is the cost, who is going to oppose effective tobacco control, and how and why—and why is what you are asking for the right thing to do.
2. Tell stories; have a clear "ask" for action to protect children and youth from tobacco and secondhand smoke
3. Build coalitions—ending addiction to nicotine and creating a tobacco-free generation is a marathon event, not a sprint.
4. Be prepared to counter industry efforts to discredit your arguments and delay or avoid effective regulation
5. Be persistent; find opportunities for success

Tobacco is the only consumer product which used as directed to kills its users. Non-smokers, and especially children, have "no voice, and no choice" in their exposure, and young people become addicted before they truly understand the long-term consequences of disease and death from tobacco. Thus, it's important for child health advocates to continue speak out and advocate for tobacco control that protects vulnerable populations—especially our children and youth.

CLINICS CARE POINTS

- Refer parents who smoke to cessation programs and advise them to limit their children's exposure to secondhand smoke exposure.

- When working with older children and adolescents, promote abstinence from smoking and all tobacco or nicotine use. Ask patients if they smoke, encourage them to remain smoke free, and counsel them to avoid secondhand smoke exposure. Remember, addiction is best prevented.

- Cessation requires chronic treatment and counseling; remain persistent when treating smokers and those attempting to quit.

DISCLOSURE

The authors have nothing to disclose.

REFERENCES

1. Musk AW, de Klerk NH. History of tobacco and health. Respirology 2003;8(3):286–90.
2. Mishra S, Mishra MB. Tobacco: Its historical, cultural, oral, and periodontal health association. J Int Soc Prev Community Dent 2013;3(1):12–8.
3. The Editors of Encyclopaedia. Jean Nicot. Britannica. https://www.britannica.com/biography/Jean-Nicot. Accessed October 17, 2022.
4. American lung association anti-spitting campaign and modern health crusade. http://exhibits.hsl.virginia.edu/alav/campaigns/. Accessed October 17, 2022.
5. Alston LJ, Dupré R, Nonnenmacher T. Social reformers and regulation: the prohibition of cigarettes in the United States and Canada. Explorations Econ Hist 2002;39(4):425–45.
6. Lombard HL, Doering CR. Cancer studies in massachusetts: habits, characteristics and environment of individuals with and without cancer. N Engl J Med 1928;198(10):481–7.
7. Pearl R. Tobacco smoking and longevity. Science 1938;87(2253):216–7.
8. Gardner MN, Brandt AM. "The doctors' choice is America's choice": the physician in US cigarette advertisements, 1930-1953. Am J Public Health 2006;96(2):222–32.
9. Klara R. Throwback Thursday: When Doctors Prescribed 'Healthy' Cigarette Brands. Adweek Web site. 2015. Available at: https://www.adweek.com/brand-marketing/throwback-thursday-when-doctors-prescribed-healthy-cigarette-brands-165404/. Accessed May 1, 2022.
10. UCSF Center for Tobacco Control Research and Education. Smoke free movies, 1920s-1950s. https://smokefreemovies.ucsf.edu/history/1920s-1950s. Accessed October 17, 2022.
11. Smith EA, Malone RE. Everywhere the soldier will be": wartime tobacco promotion in the US military. Am J Public Health 2009;99(9):1595–602.
12. Institute of Medicine. Ending the tobacco problem: a blueprint for the nation. Washington, DC: The National Academies Press; 2007.
13. Tobacco Industry Research Committee. Tobaco tactics web site. 2020. https://tobaccotactics.org/wiki/tobacco-industry-research-committee/. Accessed October 17, 2022.

14. Pollay RW, Dewhirst T. The dark side of marketing seemingly "Light" cigarettes: successful images and failed fact. Tob Control 2002;11(Suppl 1):I18–31.

15. Tobacco Institute. University of Bath. Tobacco Tactics Web site. 2020. https://tobaccotactics.org/wiki/tobacco-institute/. Accessed August 23, 2020.

16. Joseph AM, Muggli M, Pearson KC, et al. The cigarette manufacturers' efforts to promote tobacco to the U.S. military. Mil Med 2005;170(10):874–80.

17. Villanti AC, Johnson AL, Glasser AM, et al. Association of flavored tobacco use with tobacco initiation and subsequent use among US youth and adults, 2013-2015. JAMA Netw Open 2019;2(10):e1913804.

18. Huang J, Duan Z, Kwok J, et al. Vaping versus JUULing: how the extraordinary growth and marketing of JUUL transformed the US retail e-cigarette market. Tob Control 2019;28(2):146.

19. Wang TW, Trivers KF, Marynak KL, et al. Harm perceptions of intermittent tobacco product use among U.S. youth, 2016. J Adolesc Health 2018;62(6):750–3.

20. McMillen R, Klein JD, Wilson K, et al. E-cigarette use and future cigarette initiation among never smokers and relapse among former smokers in the PATH study. Public Health Rep 2019;134(5):528–36.

21. Amrock SM, Lee L, Weitzman M. Perceptions of e-cigarettes and noncigarette tobacco products among US youth. Pediatrics 2016;138(5):e20154306.

22. World Health Organization. Tobacco control in south-east asia. https://www.who.int/southeastasia/health-topics/tobacco. Accessed October 17, 2022.

23. World Health Organization. Tobacco control in south-east asia region. https://www.who.int/southeastasia/health-topics/tobacco/tobacco-control-in-the-south-east-asia-region. Accessed October 17, 2022.

24. National Cancer Institute and Centers for Disease Control and Prevention. Smokeless Tobacco and Public Health: A Global Perspective. Bethesda, MD: U.S. Department of Health and Human Services, Centers for Disease Control and Prevention and National Institutes of Health, National Cancer Institute. NIH Publication No. 14-7983; 2014.

25. World Health Organization. European tobacco use: Trends report 2019. 2019. Available at: https://www.euro.who.int/en/health-topics/disease-prevention/tobacco/publications/2019/european-tobacco-use-trends-report-2019-2019. Accessed May 2, 2022.

26. World Health Organization. Tobacco Data and Statistics. Available at: https://www.euro.who.int/en/health-topics/disease-prevention/tobacco/data-and-statistics. Accessed May 2, 2022.

27. Polanska K, Znyk M, Kaleta D. Susceptibility to tobacco use and associated factors among youth in five central and eastern European countries. BMC Public Health 2022;22(1):72.

28. Egbe CO, Magati P, Wanyonyi E, et al. Landscape of tobacco control in sub-Saharan Africa. Tob Control 2022;31(2):153–9.

29. WHO global report on trends in prevalence of tobacco smoking 2000-2025. second edition. Geneva: World Health Organization; 2018.

30. World Health Organization. Tobacco use falling: WHO urges countries to invest in helping more people to quit tobacco. 2021. https://www.who.int/news/item/16-11-2021-tobacco-use-falling-who-urges-countries-to-invest-in-helping-more-people-to-quit-tobacco. Accessed October 17, 2022.

31. Tobacco tactics: Latin America and caribbean region. University of Bath; 2021. Available at: https://tobaccotactics.org/wiki/latin-america-and-caribbean-region/. Accessed October 17, 2022.

32. Sreeramareddy CT, Pradhan PMS, Mir IA, et al. Smoking and smokeless tobacco use in nine South and Southeast Asian countries: prevalence estimates and social determinants from Demographic and Health Surveys. Popul Health Metrics 2014;12(1):22.
33. American Lung Association. 2021 federal action plan: tobacco priorities. 2021. https://www.lung.org/policy-advocacy/federal-action-plan/tobacco-priorities. Accessed October 17, 2022.
34. Mishra A, Chaturvedi P, Datta S, et al. Harmful effects of nicotine. Indian J Med Paediatr Oncol 2015;36(1):24–31.
35. Schröder R, Reuter M, Faßbender K, et al. The role of the SLC6A3 3' UTR VNTR in nicotine effects on cognitive, affective, and motor function. Psychopharmacology (Berl) 2022;239(2):489–507.
36. McGrath-Morrow SA, Gorzkowski J, Groner JA, et al. The Effects of Nicotine on Development. Pediatrics 2020;145(3).
37. Centers for Disease Control and Prevention. Smoking & tobacco use: heart disease and stroke 2020.
38. US Food & Drug Administration. How smoking affects heart health. 2021. https://www.fda.gov/tobacco-products/health-effects-tobacco-use/how-smoking-affects-heart-health. Accessed October 17, 2022.
39. National Center for Chronic Disease Prevention and Health Promotion (US) Office on Smoking and Health. The health Consequences of smoking-50 Years of progress: a Report of the Surgeon general. Atlanta (GA): Centers for Disease Control and Prevention (US); 2014.
40. Centers for Disease Control and Prevention. Health effects of cigarette smoking. 2021. https://www.cdc.gov/tobacco/data_statistics/fact_sheets/health_effects/effects_cig_smoking/index.htm. Accessed October 17, 2022.
41. Lung Cancer. https://www.wcrf.org/diet-activity-and-cancer/cancer-types/lung-cancer/. Accessed October 17, 2022.
42. Campagna D, Alamo A, Di Pino A, et al. Smoking and diabetes: dangerous liaisons and confusing relationships. Diabetol Metab Syndr 2019;11(1):85.
43. Siddiqi K, Husain S, Vidyasagaran A, et al. Global burden of disease due to smokeless tobacco consumption in adults: an updated analysis of data from 127 countries. BMC Med 2020;18(1):222.
44. Centers for Disease Control and Prevention. Tobacco industry marketing. 2021. https://www.cdc.gov/tobacco/data_statistics/fact_sheets/tobacco_industry/marketing/index.htm. Accessed October 17, 2022.
45. Kickbusch I, Allen L, Franz C. The commercial determinants of health. Lancet Glob Health 2016;4(12):e895–6.
46. World Health Organization. Tobacco: Industry tactics to attract younger generations. 2020. Available at: https://www.who.int/news-room/questions-and-answers/item/tobacco-industry-tactics-to-attract-younger-generations. Accessed May 2, 2022.
47. Riley KE, Ulrich MR, Hamann HA, et al. Decreasing Smoking but Increasing Stigma? Anti-tobacco Campaigns, Public Health, and Cancer Care. AMA J Ethics 2017;19(5):475–85.
48. Tobacco free florida. powerful anti-smoking ad campaigns work. 2022. https://tobaccofreeflorida.com/blog/powerfulads/. Accessed October 17, 2022.
49. Sandford A. Government action to reduce smoking. Respirology 2003;8(1):7–16.
50. Tobacco Twenty-One. Toabcco 21: The Law of the Land. https://tobacco21.org/. Accessed October 17, 2022.

51. Withers T., New Zealand law to ban tobacco sale to those born after 2008. Available at: https://www.bloomberg.com/news/articles/2021-12-09/new-zealand-aims-for-smokefree-generation-with-new-tobacco-law#:~:text=New%20Zealand%20Law%20to%20Ban%20Tobacco%20Sale%20to%20Those%20Born%20After%202008&text=The%20new%20law%20will%20also,to%20be%20sold%20from%202025. Accessed May 1, 2022.

52. Tobacco Free Kids. Tobacco Industry Arguments and How to Counter Them (in brief). https://www.tobaccofreekids.org/plainpackaging/intro/tobacco-industry-arguments. Accessed October 17, 2022.

53. McDaniel PA, Malone RE. Tobacco industry and public health responses to state and local efforts to end tobacco sales from 1969-2020. PLoS One 2020;15(5): e0233417.

54. Mbulo L, Palipudi KM, Andes L, et al. Secondhand smoke exposure at home among one billion children in 21 countries: findings from the Global Adult Tobacco Survey (GATS). Tob Control 2016;25(e2):e95–100.

55. Farber HJ, Walley SC, Groner JA, et al. Clinical Practice Policy To Protect Children From Tobacco, Nicotine, And Tobacco Smoke. Pediatrics 2015;136(5):1008–17.

56. Sthapit B, Chhibber, M., Twentyman, E., Naseer, S., Resnick, EA., Ahluwalia, I., Klein, JD. Maternal, newborn, and child health guidelines and tobacco control in low and lower middle income countries. APHA Annual Meeting; 2020.

57. Klein JD, Resnick EA, Chamberlin ME, Kress EA. Second-hand smoke surveillance and COVID-19: a missed opportunity. Tob Control. 2021, tobaccocontrol-2021-056532. https://doi.org/10.1136/tobaccocontrol-2021-056532.

58. Roemer R, Taylor A, Lariviere J. Origins of the WHO framework convention on tobacco control. Am J Public Health 2005;95(6):936–8.

59. WHO report on the global tobacco epidemic, 2008: the MPOWER package. Geneva: World Health Organization; 2008.

60. Global progress report on implementation of the WHO Framework Convention on Tobacco Control. Geneva: World Health Organization; 2018.

61. Perez-Warnisher MT, De Miguel M, Seijo LM. Tobacco Use Worldwide: Legislative Efforts to Curb Consumption. Ann Glob Health 2018;84(4):571–9.

62. Montini T, Bero LA. Policy makers' perspectives on tobacco control advocates' roles in regulation development. Tob Control 2001;10(3):218–24.

63. David AM, Mercado SP, Klein JD, et al. Protecting children and families from tobacco and tobacco-related NCDs in the Western Pacific: good practice examples from Malaysia, Philippines and Singapore. Child Care Health Dev 2017; 43(5):774–8.

64. American Academy of Pediatrics. Strengthening Pediatricians' Capacity for Global Tobacco Control. Available at: https://downloads.aap.org/AAP/PDF/AAP_CDC_Global_Tobacco_Fact_Sheet_2020_02.pdf. Accessed May 2, 2022.

65. World Health O, United Nations Population F, World B, United Nations Children's F. Pregnancy, childbirth, postpartum and newborn care: a guide for essential practice. 3rd ed. Geneva: World Health Organization; 2015.

66. Wilson K, Klein JD, Cowal S, et al. Addressing Tobacco And Secondhand Smoke Exposure In Maternal And Child Survival Programs. Health Affairs Blog Web site. 2015. Available at: https://www.healthaffairs.org/do/10.1377/forefront.20151124.051977. Accessed May 2, 2022.

67. Matheson I, Rivrud GN. The Effect of Smoking on Lactation and Infantile Colic. JAMA 1989;261(1):42–3.

68. Hopkinson JM, Schanler RJ, Fraley JK, et al. Milk production by mothers of premature infants: influence of cigarette smoking. Pediatrics 1992;90(6):934–8.

69. Primo CC, Ruela PBF, Brotto LDdA, et al. Effects of maternal nicotine on breast-feeding infants. Rev Paul Pediatr 2013;31(3):392–7.
70. US AID. Tobacco Policy. In US AID OPerational Policy (ADS) Series 200 Chapters. Available at: https://www.usaid.gov/sites/default/files/documents/1864/210.pdf. Accessed May 2, 2022.
71. World Health Organization. Tobacco control to improve child health and development. 2021. Available at: https://www.who.int/publications/i/item/9789240022218. Accessed May 2, 2022.

The Pediatrician's Role in Protecting Children from Environmental Hazards

Leonardo Trasande, MD, MPP[a,b,c,d,e],*,
Christopher D. Kassotis, PhD[f]

KEYWORDS

- Lead • Pesticides • Flame retardants • Endocrine disruption • Phthalates
- Bisphenols

KEY POINTS

- Children are uniquely vulnerable to a broad suite of environmental contaminants.
- Although metals and air pollutants are the focus of environmental health training in medical school and residency, endocrine disrupting chemicals have emerged as major drivers of disease and disability.
- Regulatory measures have and will continue to prove crucial in preventing diseases of environmental origin in youth.
- Anticipatory guidance in primary care settings should routinely emphasize steps families can take to limit exposures.

THE INCREASINGLY CHEMICAL WORLD EXPERIENCED BY CHILDREN

The 1993 National Academy of Sciences (NAS) report on Pesticides in the Diets of Infants and Children documented the biological basis of children's unique vulnerability to environmental hazards. Children have greater dietary intake and inhalation rates per unit body weight that magnify exposure.[2] Dermal barriers are physiologically thinner.[3] They also have more years of life in which consequences of exposure can manifest. The work of the late Sir David Barker emphasized the exquisite sensitivity of developmental programming, producing consequences for organ systems that can be permanent and lifelong.[4,5]

[a] Department of Pediatrics, Division of Environmental Pediatrics, NYU Grossman School of Medicine, New York, NY, USA; [b] Department of Population Health, NYU Grossman School of Medicine, New York, NY, USA; [c] Department of Environmental Medicine, NYU Grossman School of Medicine, New York, NY, USA; [d] NYU Wagner School of Public Service, New York, NY, USA; [e] NYU School of Global Public Health, New York, NY, USA; [f] Institute of Environmental Health Sciences and Department of Pharmacology, Wayne State University, Detroit, MI, USA
* Corresponding author. Department of Pediatrics, New York University School of Medicine, 227 East 30th Street Room 807, New York, NY 10016.
E-mail address: leonardo.trasande@nyulangone.org

Pediatr Clin N Am 70 (2023) 137–150
https://doi.org/10.1016/j.pcl.2022.09.003
0031-3955/23/© 2022 Elsevier Inc. All rights reserved.

Box 1
Selected steps that families can take to limit EDC exposures

- Avoiding microwaving food or beverages in plastic
- Eating organic
- Not cleaning plastics in the dishwasher
- Using alternatives, such as glass or stainless steel, when possible
- Avoiding plastics with recycling codes 3 (phthalates), 6 (styrene), and 7 (bisphenols) via the recycling code on the bottom of products
- Using cast iron and/or stainless steel pans instead of nonstick cooking materials
- Selecting personal care products using tools such as Environmental Working Groups' SkinDeep app
- Avoiding cleaning materials without fragrances or undisclosed ingredients
- Recirculating indoor air with outdoor air
- Using a wet mop to remove dust from electronics and furniture

---

Lead,[6–8] mercury,[9–11] tobacco smoke,[12] alcohol,[13] and polychlorinated biphenyls (PCBs)[14] were among the earliest known hazards identified in children, with consequences for cognitive impairments and other developmental disabilities.[15] Air pollutants were identified to exacerbate and induce asthma in children.[16–19] Understandably, residency programs focused training in environmental health on heavy metals and airborne contaminants.[20] The positive benefits of educational initiatives are manifest in the high self-efficacy pediatricians describe in managing lead exposures and communicating advice for prevention to families (Trasande L, Ziebold C, Schiff JS, et al. The environment in pediatric practice in Minnesota: attitudes, beliefs, and practices towards children's environmental health. Minnesota Medicine, submitted. 2008).[21–23]

However, in the 30 years since the NAS report,[1] technologic advances have further transformed the landscape of environmental exposures and identified that an even broader array of chemicals can interfere with hormone action. Endocrine-disrupting chemicals (EDCs) are ubiquitous in the human environment, and include: pharmaceuticals (eg, ethinylestradiol, rosiglitazone); ingredients in cosmetics and personal care products (eg, phthalates, parabens); pesticides, herbicides and fungicides (eg, chlorpyrifos, glyphosate); industrial chemicals (eg, bisphenols, polybrominated diphenyl ethers, PBDEs); metals (eg, arsenic, cadmium); and synthetic and naturally occurring hormones (eg, progesterone, testosterone).[24] More than 1000 chemicals have been

---

Box 2
Selected advocacy organizations leading on behalf of children's environmental health

Children's Environmental Health Network (cehn.org)

Defend Our Health (defendourhealth.org)

Endocrine Society (endocrine.org)

Environmental Working Group (ewg.org)

Food Packaging Forum (foodpackagingforum.org)

Health Care Without Harm (noharm.org)

International POPs Elimination Network (ipen.org)

identified as endocrine disruptors, including many common-use chemicals, with the vast majority of chemicals in commerce still not evaluated for EDC properties.

Health care facilities also use many products that increase the risk of EDC exposures.[25] Phthalates, for example, are abundant in polyvinylchloride-based medical devices such as blood bags, nutrition pockets, tubing, umbilical venous catheters or disposable gloves, where they can account for up to 40% of the final product by mass.[26] They are also used to make coatings for oral medications and in flooring.[27] Exposures are likely the greatest per pound body weight in neonatal intensive care units, where noninvasive respiratory support and feeding tubes have been identified as the most significant drivers of phthalate exposure.[28] In addition, bisphenols are used in polycarbonate-based medical tubing, hemodialysis equipment, newborn incubators, syringes and nebulizers.[29] Parabens are used in medications and intravenous catheters for their antimicrobial properties.[30]

The endocrine system is crucial to the functioning of nearly all human biological functions, with EDCs inducing a broad array of consequences.[31] The implications of EDCs for children's health have been codified by the World Health Organization and the United Nations Environment Program,[32] Endocrine Society,[33,34] American Academy of Pediatrics (AAP),[35] and International Federation of Obstetricians and Gynecologists (FIGO).[36] The Developmental Origins of Health and Disease hypothesis has also been expanded beyond the effects of nutritional deprivation described by Barker and colleagues[16–19] to recognize the broader range of subtler insults, including environmental exposures, which can also disrupt developmental programming.[37] The science of epigenetics has further unraveled the multigenerational consequences of environmental hazards,[38–42] and reinforced the reality that EDCs need not be structurally similar to hormones to have effects on their function.[34]

Known Effects of Environmental Hazards on Children's Health

Beginning in 1997, the NIEHS-EPA Children's Environmental Health and Disease Prevention Research Centers (Children's Centers) produced much of the direct evidence of harm induced by environmental exposures, and particularly EDCs. Multiple birth cohorts independently documented how organophosphate (OP) pesticide, and polybrominated diphenylether (PBDE) exposures resulted in consistent decrements in cognitive function in relation to prenatal exposure, controlling for multiple other potential predictors (eg, socioeconomic status and other environmental exposures); these effects are consistent with those previously observed with lead.[43–49] Specifically, prenatal exposure to OPs has been associated with magnetic resonance imaging findings in children including frontal and parietal cortical thinning that are consistent with the neurobehavioral deficits identified in psychological testing.[46]

The Children's Centers identified contributions of polycyclic aromatic hydrocarbons, traffic-related air pollution (TRAP), bisphenols and phthalates to obesity and insulin resistance in youth, independent of diet and physical activity.[50–54] These findings changed the paradigm of childhood obesity from a simple imbalance in energy consumption versus expenditure to embrace the built environment and chemicals as also being obesogenic.[50–55] Center investigators also revealed second-hand tobacco smoke, PBDEs, PAHs, and PCBs as risks for childhood leukemia,[56–58] and disruption of pubertal timing by phthalates and PBDEs.[59,60] PCBs and PBDEs were found to induce immune disruption,[61] whereas air pollution and OP exposures *in utero* were associated with increased risk for autism spectrum disorder.[62,63]

Findings from these and other studies worldwide support substantial contribution of EDCs to disease and disability in children.[24] In children born in 2010 alone, PBDE exposures in the United States accounted for 11 million IQ points lost and 43,000 cases of intellectual disability, costing $266 billion in health care and other associated costs. OP pesticide exposures accounted for another 1.8 million IQ points lost and 7500 cases of intellectual disability, costing $42 billion. Of 4-year-old children with obesity, 6.7% were attributed to prenatal bisphenol exposure, with associated costs of $2.4 billion.[64] These are an annual cost insofar as exposures continue at current levels. Importantly, these costs only accounted for the relative health impacts of a few select EDCs with substantial epidemiologic and mechanistic evidence; studies evaluating human health impacts from hundreds of other identified EDCs with known human exposures are not established enough to provide this level of evidence to calculate health costs.

The Importance of Environmental Regulation in Shaping the Health of Children

The importance of public policy in reducing children's exposure to lead is a crucial and positive example of the benefits that can be produced by protecting children from environmental hazards. Between 1976 and 1980, as the ban on lead from gasoline in the United States was being instituted, the average child blood lead level was 17.1 µg/dL among 1- to 5-year-olds. By 1999, the average had declined ~88% to 2.0 µg/dL, further fueled by bans on lead in paint. Grosse and colleagues estimate that children born in the 1990s had IQ points on average 2.2 to 4.7 IQ points higher than children born in the 1970s. The improvement in lifetime economic productivity due to these policy changes was estimated to be $110 to 319 billion annually,[65] an ongoing economic benefit that increases to this day as lead levels continue to diminish as lead-based paint hazards are eradicated. Reductions in criminality and increases in high school graduation rates have also been related to lower blood lead levels in children.[66]

Similar health and economic benefits can be traced to the 1990 Clean Air Act amendments, which strengthened federal government authority to enforce regulations that limit air pollution.[67] Between 1997 to 2008 childhood asthma morbidity declined substantially.[68] Premature births due to fine particulate matter are also likely to have declined.[69] Children from three cohorts of southern California in 2007 to 2011 were found to have greater growth in their lung function between the ages of 11 and 15 compared with similar aged populations followed between 1994 to 1998 and 1997 to 2001, due to increasingly stringent vehicle emissions limits and subsequent improvements in air quality.[70]

Ongoing Flaws in the Regulatory Framework

In the United States, chemical regulation is administered by the Environmental Protection Agency (EPA) and the Food and Drug Administration (FDA). The Toxic Substances Control Act (TSCA) provides the EPA with oversight of most commercial uses of industrial chemicals, except for pesticides. Authority for pesticide regulation is provided to EPA under the Federal Insecticide, Fungicide and Rodenticide Act and the Federal Food Drug and Cosmetic Act (FFDCA). FDA has authority to regulate chemicals used in cosmetics and personal care products, food and food packaging, and pharmaceuticals under FFDCA.

TSCA does not address EDCs or require testing for endocrine disruption, despite a revision in 2016.[71] This is problematic, as understanding of EDCs continues to accelerate rapidly, with only ~5% of synthetic chemicals tested for their potential endocrine disruption. The US FDA, for example, has now identified more than 1800 chemicals that disrupt at least one of three endocrine pathways (estrogen, androgen, and thyroid).[72]

Even if testing data are available, EPA regulatory policies continue to adhere to the Paracelsian notion that "Solely the dose determines that a thing is not a poison."

Although this adage has been fundamental to toxicologic science and in shaping regulatory policy, EDCs have revealed the flaws in the Paracelsian paradigm. EDCs are often able to promote effects at concentrations below those traditionally examined in toxicologic risk assessments.[71] They can exhibit non-monotonic dose response curves, resulting in quantitatively and qualitatively different outcomes at low versus high concentrations.[73] Greater effects have been identified during critical windows of development, with disruption during these windows altering normal development and promoting disease.[34] There is clearly a need for a shift from a flawed, risk-based paradigm to one that proactively excludes chemicals with some evidence of hazardous properties.[74]

Flaws in FDA policy frameworks also limit the capacity to address EDCs using the latest endocrine science. For example, the Food Additives Amendment of 1958 exempted food additives from regulation "if such substance is not generally recognized, among experts qualified by scientific training and experience to evaluate its safety." The Generally Recognized as Safe (GRAS) exemption has resulted in greater than 10,000 additives allowable in US food through exemptions and limits on FDA authority.[75,76] The Federal Fair Packaging and Labeling Act of 1973 initially required cosmetics ingredients to be listed on product labels, but concerns over trade secrets led to the exemption of the term "fragrance," used to describe a combination of chemicals including phthalates, solvents, preservatives, UV absorbers, and other chemical constituents known or suspected to be EDCs.[77]

In the absence of strong FDA and EPA regulatory frameworks, new chemicals have been introduced as replacements for chemicals of concern without a regulatory framework that fully evaluates their potential effects on children:

- Chemically similar bisphenols (eg, bisphenol S, or BPS) have replaced BPA;[78–83]
- Organophosphate esters (OPE) have replaced PBDEs in electronics;[84]
- Diisononylphthalate (DINP), diisodecylphthalate (DIDP) and 1,2-cyclohexane dicarboxylic acid diisononyl ester (DINCH) are replacing di-2-ethylhexylphthalate (DEHP) in food packaging;[85]
- Neonicotinoids are emerging in use as insecticides, replacing OPs and pyrethroids[86]; and
- Short-chain PFAS are increasingly replacing their long-chain analogues.[87]

Unfortunately, regrettable substitutes have been identified to produce similar effects as the chemicals they replace in all the above examples. For example, the few studies that have studied BPA replacements such as BPS have identified similar genotoxicity and estrogenicity,[78–83] embryonal effects,[88] oxidative stress,[89] cardiotoxicity,[90] disruption of osteoblast function,[91] and greater resistance to environmental degradation.[92,93]

Comparing the costs of EDCs between Europe and the United States also illustrates the crucial role of regulatory policy in shaping exposures children experience in early life and their contribution to disease burden. For example, OP-related cognitive loss ($44.7 billion) was vastly lower in the United States compared with Europe ($121 billion).[94] This divergence is likely a byproduct of the 1993 Food Quality Protection Act in the United States (which required lower allowable residues of OPs in foods) in the absence of similar activity in Europe until recently.[95] The converse is true for PBDEs due to TB-117, a California law that required addition of PBDEs to furniture from the 1970s until 2013, when the requirement was withdrawn. In contrast, Europe banned PBDEs from use much earlier, reducing the costs of exposure drastically compared with the United States.[64]

Without effective federal regulations governing EDCs, individual states have undertaken more local efforts to restrict or ban individual chemicals or classes. New York has passed a Consumer Chemical Awareness Act that notifies consumers about personal care products that contain one or more EDCs. New Jersey, New Hampshire, and Michigan have set regulations on PFAS levels in water that are considerably lower than federal limits.

Opportunities for Prevention in the Clinical Setting

Intervention studies have promise in reducing EDC exposures. Though large-scale intervention studies have not yet been conducted, small-scale interventions have supported the feasibility of reducing EDC exposures (**Boxes 1** and **2**). Lu and colleagues reduced OP metabolites in the urine of children to nondetectable levels through an organic diet intervention.[96] Though concerns about the additional costs associated with organic food are appropriate, a more recent dietary intervention also produced similar reduction in pesticide metabolites in a low-income, agricultural population.[97] A recent intervention study in young girls found that choosing personal care products that are labeled to be free of phthalates, parabens, triclosan, and benzophenones can reduce personal exposure to these EDCs by 27% to 44%.[98] Another dietary intervention study, which replaced diets in a small sample of families with fresh foods, reduced urinary levels of phthalate metabolites and bisphenols by 53% to 56%.[99]

Household interventions can also reduce exposure. A recent study measured dust from offices, common areas, and classrooms having undergone no intervention (conventional rooms in older buildings meeting strict fire codes), full "healthier" materials interventions (rooms with "healthier" materials in buildings constructed more recently or gut-renovated), or partial interventions (other rooms with at least "healthier" foam furniture but more potential building contamination). Rooms with full "healthier" materials interventions had 78% lower dust levels of PFAS than rooms with no intervention ($P < 0.01$). Rooms with full "healthier" interventions also had 65% lower OPE levels in dust than rooms with no intervention ($P < 0.01$) and 45% lower PBDEs than rooms with only partial interventions ($P < 0.1$), adjusted for covariates related to insulation, electronics, and furniture.[100]

It should be noted that not all studies have achieved expected changes in EDC levels. One study reported an increase in urinary phthalate metabolites in the intervention group, which was determined to be due to substantial phthalate contamination in the coriander provided to participants.[101] Another more recent study attempted to create a BPA risk score based on characteristics of food containers and packaging, and was unable to reduce urinary levels.[102]

Though further research is particularly needed to generalize the interventions which have been shown to reduce exposure, the American Academy of Pediatrics (AAP) Council on Environmental Health has published multiple policy statements on pesticides[103] and chemicals intentionally and unintentionally added to foods.[35] The AAP guidance suggests reductions in exposure to pesticides in foods, and identifies steps including the consumption of organic produce, recognizing the nutritional, environmental, health and cost issues involved. It documents the variability of pesticide residues, as they are highest in leafy fruits and vegetables, and refers to various guides provided by Consumer Reports (Stop Eating Pesticides) and Environmental Working Group (Dirty Dozen and Clean Fifteen lists). Rinsing fruits can reduce residues but has not been proven to reduce exposure.[104]

The Importance of the Pediatrician Voice in Environmental Advocacy

The medical professional community has called their members to action to protect their patients from EDC exposure, including (but not limited to) the American Academy of Pediatrics,[35] Endocrine Society,[33,34] and International Federation of Obstetricians and Gynecologists.[36] This section describes patient- and government-level advocacy opportunities for pediatricians steeped in the latest scientific evidence.

The AAP Policy Statement on Pesticides recommends improved labeling on pesticide containers including inert ingredients and risks posed specifically to children. It also supports improved reporting requirements for poisonings, and the support of least toxic alternatives, including the use of integrated pest management in households and agricultural settings, both in the United States and abroad. The Policy Statement also endorses the notion that communities and its members have the right to know where pesticides are applied, so that modifications can be made to reduce exposures in vulnerable groups.[105]

The AAP Policy Statement on Food Additive Chemicals identifies multiple improvements needed in FFDCA reform, including:

- Revising the GRAS process permit independent scientific review, followed by FDA review of such evaluations, before approval;
- Eliminating conflicts of interest in toxicologic evaluations of food additives;
- Requiring FDA to consider vulnerable subpopulations and systems in evaluating food additive safety, and applying additional safety factors to account for this vulnerability;
- Considering cumulative exposure from all dietary sources, as well as other additives and contaminants that interact with the same biological pathways; and
- Expanded FDA authority to revisit safety of chemicals when concerns are raised.

The Endocrine Society has also called for a shift from a flawed, risk-based paradigm to one that proactively excludes chemicals with some evidence of hazardous properties until further detailed reassuring testing data become available.[74] This call is based upon growing evidence that EDCs can exhibit nonlinear and non-monotonic dose response curves, resulting in quantitatively and qualitatively different outcomes at low versus high concentrations.[73] This phenomenon means that effects of low-level exposures in humans cannot be extrapolated from high-dose experiments in animals, leaving to a false interpretation of safety.[34]

Health care facilities have also begun to support sustainability initiatives that reduce the use of plastic, particularly those with chemical hazards. Practice Greenhealth, a network of over 1,400 hospitals in the United States, has implemented sustainability initiatives and climate-smart strategies in their facilities. The network also includes industry partners (manufacturers, suppliers, service providers, and other supply chain partners). Health Care without Harm supports hospital partners in recommending safer medical products and other materials that health care organizations and hospitals should adopt.

ADVOCATING FOR MEDICAL EDUCATIONAL CHANGE

Rapidly accelerating awareness about the threat of climate change, especially among medical students and residents, has brought to the fore the need for enhanced environmental health education in the medical curriculum. Given that many EDCs derive from fossil fuels, there are potential co-benefits to reductions in their production. Increasing awareness of these exposures among the public also raises the need for educational efforts that span the population of child health care providers from pediatric interns to senior practitioners.

The surveys of state chapter membership of the AAP in Michigan,[106] Minnesota, (Trasande L, Ziebold C, Schiff JS, et al. The environment in pediatric practice in Minnesota: attitudes, beliefs, and practices towards children's environmental health.

Minnesota Medicine, submitted. 2008.)Wisconsin[23] and New York,[21] which revealed strong self-efficacy in managing lead exposure, also identified a lack of self-efficacy in managing patients with pesticide and other EDC exposures (and supporting anticipatory guidance around prevention). These findings were also confirmed among obstetricians and gynecologists.[107] Gaps in provider self-efficacy related to managing EDCs should not be surprising given the limited amount of environmental health education in medical training.[108] A survey of pediatric residencies in 2003 revealed a modest (typically 1–6 hour) focus on environmental hazards across 3-year programs. Clearly, there is a need for updating medical school curricula.

To address gaps in active practitioners, the Endocrine Society has organized a series of educational videos for health care providers, now posted on YouTube and the Endocrine Society website (www.endocrine.org). The International Federation of Gynecologists and Obstetricians has also developed a series of patient-facing materials to guide families about safe and simple steps to reduce exposure. The Council on Environmental Health of the AAP has produced patient- and provider-facing educational materials linked to the pesticide and food additive statements. Each of these initiatives represents an important advance in our ability to protect children.

Pediatricians have long served as outstanding advocates, from childhood vaccines to injury prevention. Although EDCs and other environmental exposures compete for attention with other aspects of anticipatory guidance, as well as treatment for acute conditions, their increasing contribution to chronic diseases that increasingly affect youth cannot be neglected. The best treatment will ultimately come from primary prevention of toxic exposures, through the combination of individual- and population-level advocacy. The voice of the pediatrician remains extremely well-respected in both of these circles, and given the known contribution of these exposures to disease and disability across the lifespan, we all stand to benefit when pediatricians show true leadership on behalf of the most vulnerable.

DISCLOSURE

L. Trasande acknowledges honoraria from Houghton Mifflin Harcourt, Audible, Paidos and Kobunsha; travel support from the Endocrine Society, WHO, UNEP, Japan Environment and Health Ministries and the American Academy of Pediatrics; as well as scientific advisory board activities for Beautycounter, IS-Global and Footprint grant P2CES033423 from National Institute of Environmental Health Sciences.

REFERENCES

1. National Research Council. Pesticides in the diets of Infants and children. Washington, DC: National Academy Press; 1993.
2. Choi J, Knudsen LE, Mizrak S, et al. Identification of exposure to environmental chemicals in children and older adults using human biomonitoring data sorted by age: Results from a literature review. Int J Hyg Environ Health 2017;220(2 Pt A):282–98.
3. Johnson-Restrepo B, Kannan K. An assessment of sources and pathways of human exposure to polybrominated diphenyl ethers in the United States. Chemosphere 2009;76(4):542–8.
4. Barker DJ, Godfrey KM, Osmond C, et al. The relation of fetal length, ponderal index and head circumference to blood pressure and the risk of hypertension in adult life. Paediatric perinatal Epidemiol 1992;6(1):35–44.
5. Barker DJ, Osmond C, Forsen TJ, et al. Trajectories of growth among children who have coronary events as adults. N Engl J Med 2005;353(17):1802–9.

6. Jusko TA, Henderson CR, Lanphear BP, et al. Blood Lead Concentrations< 10 mug/dL and Child Intelligence at 6 Years of Age. Environ Health Perspect 2008;116(2):243.

7. Lanphear B, Hornung R, Khoury J, et al. Low-level environmental lead exposure and children's intellectual function: an international pooled analysis. Environ Health Perspect 2005;113:894–9.

8. Canfield RL, Henderson CR Jr, Cory-Slechta DA, et al. Intellectual Impairment in Children with Blood Lead Concentrations below 10 {micro} g per Deciliter. N Engl J Med 2003;348(16):1517.

9. Trasande L, Landrigan PJ, Schechter C. Public health and economic consequences of methyl mercury toxicity to the developing brain. Environ Health Perspect 2005;113(5):590–6.

10. Grandjean P, Budtz-Jorgensen E, White RF, et al. Methylmercury Exposure Biomarkers as Indicators of Neurotoxicity in Children Aged 7 Years. Am J Epidemiol 2003;150:301–5.

11. National Research Council. Toxicological effects of methylmercury. Washington, DC: National Academy Press; 2000.

12. Weitzman M, Gortmaker S, Walker DK, et al. Maternal smoking and childhood asthma. Pediatrics 1990;85(4):505–11.

13. Lupton C, Burd L, Harwood R. Cost of fetal alcohol spectrum disorders. Am J Med Genet 2004;127(1):42–50.

14. Jacobson JL, Jacobson SW. Intellectual Impairment in Children Exposed to Polychlorinated Biphenyls in Utero. N Engl J Med 1996;335(11):783.

15. Trasande L. Environmental contributors to autism: the pediatrician's role. Curr Probl Pediatr Adolesc Health Care 2014;44(10):319–20.

16. McConnell R, Islam T, Shankardass K, et al. Childhood incident asthma and traffic-related air pollution at home and school. Environ Health Perspect 2010; 118(7):1021–6.

17. Trasande L, Thurston GD. The role of air pollution in asthma and other pediatric morbidities. J Allergy Clin Immunol 2005;115(4):689–99.

18. Gent JF, Triche EW, Holford TR, et al. Association of low-level ozone and fine particles with respiratory symptoms in children with asthma. JAMA 2003;290(14): 1859–67. Am Med Assoc.

19. McConnell R, Berhane K, Gilliland F, et al. Asthma in exercising children exposed to ozone: a cohort study. The Lancet 2002;359(9304):386–91.

20. Roberts JR, Gitterman BA. Pediatric environmental health education: a survey of US pediatric residency programs. Ambul Pediatr 2003;3(1):57–9.

21. Trasande L, Boscarino J, Graber N, et al. The environment in pediatric practice: a study of New York pediatricians' attitudes, beliefs, and practices towards children's environmental health. J Urban Health 2006;83(4):760–72.

22. Trasande L, Niu J, Li J, et al. The Environment and Children's Health Care in Northwest China. BMC Pediatr 2014;14:82.

23. Trasande L, Schapiro ML, Falk R, et al. Pediatrician attitudes, clinical activities, and knowledge of environmental health in Wisconsin. WMJ 2006;105(2):45–9.

24. Kahn LG, Philippat C, Nakayama SF, et al. Endocrine-disrupting chemicals: implications for human health. Lancet Diabetes Endocrinol 2020;8(8):703–18.

25. Genco M, Anderson-Shaw L, Sargis RM. Unwitting Accomplices: Endocrine Disruptors Confounding Clinical Care. J Clin Endocrinol Metab 2020;105(10): e3822–7.

26. Marie C, Hamlaoui S, Bernard L, et al. Exposure of hospitalised pregnant women to plasticizers contained in medical devices. BMC women's health 2017;17(1):45.

27. Kelley KE, Hernández-Díaz S, Chaplin EL, et al. Identification of phthalates in medications and dietary supplement formulations in the United States and Canada. Environ Health Perspect 2012;120(3):379–84.

28. Stroustrup A, Bragg JB, Busgang SA, et al. Sources of clinically significant neonatal intensive care unit phthalate exposure. J Expo Sci Environ Epidemiol 2020;30(1):137–48.

29. Bacle A, Thevenot S, Grignon C, et al. Determination of bisphenol A in water and the medical devices used in hemodialysis treatment. Int J pharmaceutics 2016; 505(1–2):115–21.

30. Shenep LE, Shenep MA, Cheatham W, et al. Efficacy of intravascular catheter lock solutions containing preservatives in the prevention of microbial colonization. J Hosp Infect 2011;79(4):317–22.

31. Ghassabian A, Vandenberg L, Kannan K, et al. Endocrine-disrupting chemicals child health. Annu Rev Pharmacol Toxicol 2022;62:573–94.

32. Bergman A, Heindel JJ, Jobling S, et al. State of the science of endocrine disrupting chemicals 2012. United National Environment Programme and Worl Health Organization; 2013.

33. Diamanti-Kandarakis E, Bourguignon J-P, Giudice LC, et al. Endocrine-Disrupting Chemicals: An Endocrine Society Scientific Statement. Endocr Rev 2009; 30(4):293–342.

34. Gore AC, Chappell VA, Fenton SE, et al. EDC-2: The Endocrine Society's Second Scientific Statement on Endocrine-Disrupting Chemicals. Endocr Rev 2015;36(6):E1–150.

35. Trasande L, Shaffer RM, Sathyanarayana S. Food Additives and Child Health. Pediatrics 2018;142(2).

36. Di Renzo GC, Conry JA, Blake J, et al. International Federation of Gynecology and Obstetrics opinion on reproductive health impacts of exposure to toxic environmental chemicals. Int J Gynecol Obstet 2015;131(3):219–25.

37. Heindel JJ, Balbus J, Birnbaum L, et al. Developmental Origins of Health and Disease: Integrating Environmental Influences. Endocrinology 2015;156(10): 3416–21.

38. Stel J, Legler J. The Role of Epigenetics in the Latent Effects of Early Life Exposure to Obesogenic Endocrine Disrupting Chemicals. Endocrinology 2015; 156(10):3466–72.

39. Skinner MK, Manikkam M, Tracey R, et al. Ancestral dichlorodiphenyltrichloroethane (DDT) exposure promotes epigenetic transgenerational inheritance of obesity. BMC Med 2013;11:228.

40. Janesick A, Blumberg B. Endocrine disrupting chemicals and the developmental programming of adipogenesis and obesity. Birth Defects Res C: Embryo Today Rev 2011;93(1):34–50.

41. Nomura T. Transgenerational carcinogenesis: induction and transmission of genetic alterations and mechanisms of carcinogenesis. Mutat Research/Reviews Mutat Res 2003;544(2):425–32.

42. Janesick AS, Shioda T, Blumberg B. Transgenerational inheritance of prenatal obesogen exposure. Mol Cell Endocrinol 2014;398(1–2):31–5.

43. Herbstman JB, Sjodin A, Kurzon M, et al. Prenatal exposure to PBDEs and neurodevelopment. Environ Health Perspect 2010;118(5):712–9.

44. Rauh VA, Garfinkel R, Perera FP, et al. Impact of prenatal chlorpyrifos exposure on neurodevelopment in the first 3 years of life among inner-city children. Pediatrics 2006;118.

45. Rauh V, Arunajadai S, Horton M, et al. Seven-year neurodevelopmental scores and prenatal exposure to chlorpyrifos, a common agricultural pesticide. Environ Health Perspect 2011;119:1196.

46. Rauh VA, Perera FP, Horton MK, et al. Brain anomalies in children exposed prenatally to a common organophosphate pesticide. Proc Natl Acad Sci U S A 2012;109(20):7871–6.

47. Engel SM, Bradman A, Wolff MS, et al. Prenatal Organophosphorus Pesticide Exposure and Child Neurodevelopment at 24 Months: An Analysis of Four Birth Cohorts. Environ Health Perspect 2015;124(6):822–30.

48. Bouchard M, Chevrier J, Harley K, et al. Prenatal exposure to organophosphate pesticides and IQ in 7-year-old children. Environ Health Perspect 2011;119:1189.

49. Engel S, Wetmur J, Chen J, et al. Prenatal exposure to organophosphates, paraoxonase 1, and cognitive development in childhood. Environ Health Perspect 2011;119:1182.

50. Rundle A, Hoepner L, Hassoun A, et al. Association of childhood obesity with maternal exposure to ambient air polycyclic aromatic hydrocarbons during pregnancy. Am J Epidemiol 2012;175(11):1163–72.

51. Harley KG, Aguilar Schall R, Chevrier J, et al. Prenatal and postnatal bisphenol A exposure and body mass index in childhood in the CHAMACOS cohort. Environ Health Perspect 2013;121(4):514–20, 520e511-516.

52. Hoepner LA, Whyatt RM, Widen EM, et al. Bisphenol A and Adiposity in an Inner-City Birth Cohort. Environ Health Perspect 2016;124(10):1644–50.

53. Buckley JP, Engel SM, Braun JM, et al. Prenatal Phthalate Exposures and Body Mass Index Among 4- to 7-Year-old Children: A Pooled Analysis. Epidemiology 2016;27(3):449–58.

54. Harley KG, Berger K, Rauch S, et al. Association of prenatal urinary phthalate metabolite concentrations and childhood BMI and obesity. Pediatr Res 2017; 82(3):405–15.

55. Maresca MM, Hoepner LA, Hassoun A, et al. Prenatal Exposure to Phthalates and Childhood Body Size in an Urban Cohort. Environ Health Perspect 2016; 124(4):514–20.

56. Deziel NC, Rull RP, Colt JS, et al. Polycyclic aromatic hydrocarbons in residential dust and risk of childhood acute lymphoblastic leukemia. Environ Res 2014;133: 388–95.

57. Gunier RB, Kang A, Hammond SK, et al. A task-based assessment of parental occupational exposure to pesticides and childhood acute lymphoblastic leukemia. Environ Res 2017;156:57–62.

58. Ward MH, Colt JS, Deziel NC, et al. Residential levels of polybrominated diphenyl ethers and risk of childhood acute lymphoblastic leukemia in California. Environ Health Perspect 2014;122(10):1110–6.

59. Wolff MS, Teitelbaum SL, McGovern K, et al. Phthalate exposure and pubertal development in a longitudinal study of US girls. Hum Reprod (Oxford, England) 2014;29(7):1558–66.

60. Harley KG, Rauch SA, Chevrier J, et al. Association of prenatal and childhood PBDE exposure with timing of puberty in boys and girls. Environ Int 2017;100: 132–8.

61. Ashwood P, Schauer J, Pessah IN, et al. Preliminary evidence of the in vitro effects of BDE-47 on innate immune responses in children with autism spectrum disorders. J neuroimmunology 2009;208(1–2):130–5.

62. Shelton JF, Geraghty EM, Tancredi DJ, et al. Neurodevelopmental disorders and prenatal residential proximity to agricultural pesticides: the CHARGE study. Environ Health Perspect 2014;122(10):1103–9.

63. Volk HE, Hertz-Picciotto I, Delwiche L, et al. Residential proximity to freeways and autism in the CHARGE study. Environ Health Perspect 2011;119(6):873–7.

64. Attina TM, Hauser R, Sathyanarayana S, et al. Exposure to endocrine-disrupting chemicals in the USA: a population-based disease burden and cost analysis. Lancet Diabetes Endocrinol 2016;4(12):996–1003.

65. Grosse SD, Matte TD, Schwartz J, et al. Economic Gains Resulting from the Reduction in Children's Exposure to Lead in the United States. Environ Health Perspect 2002;110(6):563–9.

66. Muennig P. The social costs of childhood lead exposure in the post-lead regulation era. Arch Pediatr Adolesc Med 2009;163(9):844–9.

67. Ross K, Chmiel JF, Ferkol T. The impact of the Clean Air Act. J Pediatr 2012; 161(5):781–6.

68. Trasande L, Liu Y. Reducing The Staggering Costs Of Environmental Disease In Children, Estimated At $76.6 Billion In 2008. Health Aff 2011;30(5):863–70.

69. Trasande L, Malecha P, Attina TM. Particulate Matter Exposure and Preterm Birth: Estimates of U.S. Attributable Burden and Economic Costs. Environ Health Perspect 2016;124(12):1913–8.

70. Gauderman WJ, Avol E, Gilliland F, et al. The Effect of Air Pollution on Lung Development from 10 to 18 Years of Age. N Engl J Med 2004;351(11):1057–67.

71. Kassotis CD, Trasande L. Endocrine disruptor global policy. Adv Pharmacol (San Diego, Calif) 2021;92:1–34.

72. Ding D, Xu L, Fang H, et al. The EDKB: an established knowledge base for endocrine disrupting chemicals. BMC Bioinformatics 2010;11(Suppl 6):S5.

73. Vandenberg LN, Colborn T, Hayes TB, et al. Hormones and endocrine-disrupting chemicals: low-dose effects and nonmonotonic dose responses. Endocr Rev 2012;33(3):378–455.

74. Kassotis CD, Vandenberg LN, Demeneix BA, et al. Endocrine-disrupting chemicals: economic, regulatory, and policy implications. Lancet Diabetes Endocrinol 2020;8(8):719–30.

75. Neltner TG, Alger HM, Leonard JE, et al. Data gaps in toxicity testing of chemicals allowed in food in the United States. Reprod Toxicol 2013;42(0):85–94.

76. Neltner TG, Kulkarni NR, Alger HM, et al. Navigating the U.S. Food Additive Regulatory Program. Compr Rev Food Sci Food Saf 2011;10(6):342–68.

77. Sarantis H, Naidenko OV, Gray S, et al. Not so sexy: The health risks of secret chemicals in fragrance. 2010. https://www.ewg.org/sites/default/files/report/SafeCosmetics_FragranceRpt.pdf (21 February 2022. Accessed February 21, 2022.

78. Kuruto-Niwa R, Nozawa R, Miyakoshi T, et al. Estrogenic activity of alkylphenols, bisphenol S, and their chlorinated derivatives using a GFP expression system. Environ Toxicol Pharmacol 2005;19(1):121–30.

79. Chen M-Y, Ike M, Fujita M. Acute toxicity, mutagenicity, and estrogenicity of bisphenol-A and other bisphenols. Environ Toxicol 2002;17(1):80–6.

80. Si Yoshihara, Mizutare T, Makishima M, et al. Potent Estrogenic Metabolites of Bisphenol A and Bisphenol B Formed by Rat Liver S9 Fraction: Their Structures and Estrogenic Potency. Toxicol Sci 2004;78(1):50–9.

81. Okuda K, Fukuuchi T, Takiguchi M, et al. Novel Pathway of Metabolic Activation of Bisphenol A-Related Compounds for Estrogenic Activity. Drug Metab Dispos 2011;39(9):1696–703.

82. Audebert M, Dolo L, Perdu E, et al. Use of the γH2AX assay for assessing the genotoxicity of bisphenol A and bisphenol F in human cell lines. Arch Toxicol 2011;85(11):1463–73.

83. Vinas R, Watson CS. Bisphenol S disrupts estradiol-induced nongenomic signaling in a rat pituitary cell line: effects on cell functions. Environ Health Perspect 2013;121:352–8.

84. Yang J, Zhao Y, Li M, et al. A Review of a Class of Emerging Contaminants: The Classification, Distribution, Intensity of Consumption, Synthesis Routes, Environmental Effects and Expectation of Pollution Abatement to Organophosphate Flame Retardants (OPFRs). Int J Mol Sci 2019;20(12):2874.

85. Kunikane H, Watanabe K, Fukuoka M, et al. Double-blind randomized control trial of the effect of recombinant human erythropoietin on chemotherapy-induced anemia in patients with non-small cell lung cancer. Int J Clin Oncol 2001;6(6):296–301.

86. Goulson D. REVIEW: An overview of the environmental risks posed by neonicotinoid insecticides. J Appl Ecol 2013;50(4):977–87.

87. Brendel S, Fetter É, Staude C, et al. Short-chain perfluoroalkyl acids: environmental concerns and a regulatory strategy under REACH. Environ Sci Eur 2018;30(1):9.

88. Qiu W, Zhao Y, Yang M, et al. Actions of Bisphenol A and Bisphenol S on the Reproductive Neuroendocrine System During Early Development in Zebrafish. Endocrinology 2015;157(2):636–47.

89. Zhao C, Tang Z, Yan J, et al. Bisphenol S exposure modulate macrophage phenotype as defined by cytokines profiling, global metabolomics and lipidomics analysis. Sci Total Environ 2017;592:357–65.

90. Gu J, Wang H, Zhou L, et al. Oxidative stress in bisphenol AF-induced cardiotoxicity in zebrafish and the protective role of N-acetyl N-cysteine. Sci total Environ 2020;731:139190.

91. Chin K-Y, Pang K-L, Mark-Lee WF. A Review on the Effects of Bisphenol A and Its Derivatives on Skeletal Health. Int J Med Sci 2018;15(10):1043–50.

92. Danzl E, Sei K, Soda S, et al. Biodegradation of bisphenol A, bisphenol F and bisphenol S in seawater. Int J Environ Res Public Health 2009;6(4):1472–84.

93. Ike M, Chen MY, Danzl E, et al. Biodegradation of a variety of bisphenols under aerobic and anaerobic conditions. Water Sci Technol 2006;53(6):153–9.

94. Bellanger M, Demeneix B, Grandjean P, et al. Neurobehavioral deficits, diseases, and associated costs of exposure to endocrine-disrupting chemicals in the European union. J Clin Endocrinol Metab 2015;100(4):1256–66.

95. Trasande L. When enough data are not enough to enact policy: The failure to ban chlorpyrifos. PLOS Biol 2017;15(12):e2003671.

96. Lu C, Toepel K, Irish R, et al. Organic Diets Significantly Lower Children's Dietary Exposure to Organophosphorus Pesticides. Environ Health Perspect 2006;114(2):260–3.

97. Bradman A, Quirós-Alcalá L, Castorina R, et al. Effect of Organic Diet Intervention on Pesticide Exposures in Young Children Living in Low-Income Urban and Agricultural Communities. Environ Health Perspect 2015;123(10):1086–93.

98. Harley KG, Kogut K, Madrigal DS, et al. Reducing Phthalate, Paraben, and Phenol Exposure from Personal Care Products in Adolescent Girls: Findings

from the HERMOSA Intervention Study. Environ Health Perspect 2016;124(10): 1600–7.

99. Rudel RA, Gray JM, Engel CL, et al. Food Packaging and Bisphenol A and Bis(2-Ethyhexyl) Phthalate Exposure: Findings from a Dietary Intervention. Environ Health Perspect 2011;119(7).

100. Young AS, Hauser R, James-Todd TM, et al. Impact of "healthier" materials interventions on dust concentrations of per- and polyfluoroalkyl substances, polybrominated diphenyl ethers, and organophosphate esters. Environment International; 2020. p. 106151.

101. Sathyanarayana S, Alcedo G, Saelens BE, et al. Unexpected results in a randomized dietary trial to reduce phthalate and bisphenol A exposures. J Expo Sci Environ Epidemiol 2013;23(4):378–84.

102. Galloway TS, Baglin N, Lee BP, et al. An engaged research study to assess the effect of a 'real-world' dietary intervention on urinary bisphenol A (BPA) levels in teenagers. BMJ Open 2018;8(2):e018742.

103. Forman J, Silverstein J. Organic foods: health and environmental advantages and disadvantages. Pediatrics 2012;130(5):e1406–15.

104. Krol WJ, Arsenault TL, Pylypiw HM, et al. Reduction of Pesticide Residues on Produce by Rinsing. J Agric Food Chem 2000;48(10):4666–70.

105. Council On Environmental H, Roberts JR, Karr CJ, et al. Pesticide Exposure in Children. Pediatrics 2012;130(6):e1757–63.

106. Trasande L, Newman N, Long L, et al. Translating Knowledge About Environmental Health to Practitioners: Are We Doing Enough? Mount Sinai J Med A J Translational Personalized Med 2010;77(1):114–23.

107. Stotland NE, Sutton P, Trowbridge J, et al. Counseling patients on preventing prenatal environmental exposures - a mixed-methods study of obstetricians. PLoS One 2014;9(6):e98771.

108. McCurdy LE, Roberts J, Rogers B, et al. Incorporating Environ Health into Pediatr Med Nurs Education 2004;112(17):1755–60.

Advocacy to Action

Translating Research into Child Health Policy

Aligning Incentives and Building a New Discourse

Christian D. Pulcini, MD, MEd, MPH[a],*, Jean L. Raphael, MD, MPH[b],
Keila N. Lopez, MD, MPH[b]

KEYWORDS

- Pediatrics • Research • Health policy • Evidence translation • Policy implementation
- Population health

KEY POINTS

- Translating research into policy is imperative to making impactful and sustainable improvements to the health of children and requires understanding the role and impact of the political determinants of health, structural determinants of health, social determinants of health, and health care delivery.
- Limited data on long-term return on investment, insufficient funding of research, lack of incentives for researchers to engage with policymakers, and traditionally slow dissemination of scientific information are major factors that have contributed to the pediatric evidence-policy gap.
- Multiple child health policy initiatives exist which align with the current evidence (human papilloma virus immunization), as well as those that lie in direct opposition to current evidence (childhood poverty).
- Concrete strategies are available to assist pediatric researchers in translating their research to policy, but a collaborative, supported, and concerted approach is needed by engaged key stakeholders throughout in the process.

BACKGROUND

In 2001, the Institute of Medicine, currently known as the National Academy of Medicine, published an impactful study describing the estimated lag of 17 years between when health scientists disseminate rigorous research and when health practitioners change their patient care as a result.[1] Although over 20 years have passed since

---

[a] Department of Emergency Medicine and Pediatrics, University of Vermont Larner College of Medicine, Fletcher House 301, 111 Colchester Avenue, Burlington, VT 05401, USA;
[b] Department of Pediatrics, Baylor College of Medicine, One Baylor Plaza, Houston, TX 77030, USA
* Corresponding author.
E-mail address: christian.pulcini@uvm.edu

Pediatr Clin N Am 70 (2023) 151–164
https://doi.org/10.1016/j.pcl.2022.09.012
0031-3955/23/© 2022 Elsevier Inc. All rights reserved.

this study was published, this problem has continued to plague health care systems. Compounding this evidence-to-practice gap, there is an increased recognition of the importance for academic institutions to extend research findings beyond the "ivory tower," and further, to disseminate the research to policy makers to impact meaningful health-related legislation at the local, state, and federal levels.[2]

Public policies can be impacted by basic and clinical research findings, and research priorities and funding can be impacted by public policy.[3] Thus, it is important to realize that translating research into policy is imperative to making impactful and sustainable improvements to the health of Americans.[4] However, research is limited by the amount of funding attached, time available for those to participate, and community involvement and engagement. Moreover, scaling up from a smaller successful research study that works for one population to a larger population-level intervention may not work because of a multitude of issues including non-sustainable funding and lack of generalizability. It is this translation of research into policy that ultimately impacts large populations and changes health outcomes.

Research can impact health-related policy through several avenues:

- Accurately documenting the existence, quantifying the extent, and demonstrating the correlates of a problem
- Analyzing the problem to identify what interventions work and which do not
- Identifying undesired and unintended consequences of policy decisions
- Suggesting or prescribing options to address the problem
- Raising the quality of the debate about health issues to include scholarly evidence as well as anecdotes and biases.[5]

The worlds of research and health policy often have challenges talking to each other, however, as research findings are not easily accessed by policy makers and are additionally laden with technical jargon, complex statistical models, and associations rather than the clear cause and effect conclusions with specific policy recommendations.[6]

There are examples in the last few decades of translating research into public policy in the pediatric space, including research demonstrating the association of infants safe sleeping and suddent infant death syndrome (SIDS) deaths which launched the "back to sleep" campaign. This evidence-based initiative ultimately reduced SIDS deaths by greater than 70%. Another successful example is state mandates for human papilloma virus vaccination which have reduced cervical cancer rates by nearly 90%.[7] There remains a significant amount of needed progress, however, in other areas where translation has not occurred.

Using the example of the research-to-policy gap in meaningfully addressing health disparities, as health care workers and researchers, we need to critically question how social determinants shape health and what shapes these social determinants? Further, how can we implement and translate strategies to address health inequities that we know exist? These questions require researchers to become more politically astute and pay more attention to political determinants of health (PDOH): analyzing how different power constellations, institutions, processes, interests, and ideological positions affect health within different political systems and cultures and at different levels of governance.[8,9] The PDOH are imperative to understand how population health policies are to be successfully formulated and implemented. As pediatric health researchers, it is crucial to create shared, accessible content based on our research findings that allows for quicker dissemination and adoption by our contemporaries in governance, advocacy, and policymaking to more effectively impact patient care and child health. To move toward this goal, we summarize barriers in translation of research into policy, provide examples of discordance between evidence and policy, describe current models on how to translate research to policy, and provide an agenda for translation.

THE RESEARCH TO POLICY GAP

Maximizing the impact of scientific findings requires that research be communicated effectively and efficiently to policy makers and varied invested stakeholders. A large number of studies and systematic reviews have explored barriers to translating research findings into policy.[10–15] The authors review the major factors which impede uptake of research toward policy implementation.

Return on Investment in Child Health Policy

Translating research to policy for children is critically important given strong evidence that early investments can impact children's development and their long-term ability to thrive and grow into healthy adults. However, children are frequently marginalized or altogether excluded in policy investments because financing for initiatives relies calculations of relatively short-term return on investment (ROI) within the health sector.[16] Child health policy initiatives will produce health-related financial returns, but the ROI typically occurs on a longer time horizon and likely includes savings outside the health care sector, in what is typically deemed the "wrong pockets" problem.[17] This phenomenon arises when one entity makes an investment in an initiative that, if successful, produces benefit for another entity. For example, a health policy strategy implemented to address child behavioral health may generate financial benefits that may be experienced by the education or juvenile justice systems rather than health care. The "wrong pockets" problem represents a challenge to health policy makers as it may impact sound decision-making on child health policy investments.

Pediatric Research Funding

The availability of research funding is essential to generating data that can inform policy. The National Institutes of Health (NIH) represents the largest funding source for biomedical research in the world with a budget of over $40 billion in 2020.[18] The Eunice Kennedy Shriver National Institute of Child Health and Human Development is the largest federal funding source for pediatric research. NIH-funded research programs have led to substantial improvements in pediatric health outcomes in the areas of infant and child mortality, serious pediatric infection, and neonatal care.[19] However, public investments in pediatric research have been relatively small compared with research on adults.[18,20] Investments in pediatric research have been limited by challenges in the research itself—ethical considerations regarding minors and logistical and technical factors (eg, drugs with liquid formulations). Private or commercial investments have also limited investments in pediatric research given the small market shares for pediatric drugs relative to adult drugs.[20] Consequently, fewer studies are conducted in children, the pediatric population tends to be underrepresented in randomized clinical trials, and research in certain pediatric conditions is substantially underfunded.[18,21] Relatively anemic investments in pediatric research as a whole create a multilayered pipeline problem in both the available pediatric studies that can influence policy and the sustainability of the workforce who want to do the research.

Academic Incentives and Approach to Knowledge Translation

Academic researchers exist in an environment largely built on traditional scholarly productivity incentivized toward peer-reviewed articles in scientific journals, grant procurement, and presentations in academic settings.[22] These milestones represent the currency needed to propel professional development and academic promotion. By their very nature, these milestones in academia create misalignment in translation of research into policy. Academic researchers may interpret their professional roles as very narrowly focused on generation and dissemination of scholarship as they are not judged by the impact of their research on people's lives. Their research may reflect the intellectual interests of scientists or funders and not be framed to address the priorities of policy makers. For a subset of researchers, the culture and performance metrics of academic life may even foster a risk-averse approach to knowledge generation and dissemination. In extreme cases, the paramount needs for grants and publications may lead to incremental approaches to research, overreliance on funder priorities for determining scientific directions, and focus on scholarship that is relatively easier to publish. As a result of academic incentives, the time horizon for knowledge generation and translation can be long and policy-relevant research findings may lag within the social and professional networks of academia.[23–25]

In addition to potentially perverse incentives in academia, relatively limited incorporation of stakeholder engagement into research may also hinder translation of research into policy.[26] In much of academic research, stakeholders (eg, children and families, clinicians, employers, payers, community organizations, foundations) are not routinely involved in the creation of the research project, strategies for recruitment and retention of subjects, or dissemination planning. Involvement of stakeholders in current practice may consist of limited key informant interviews or focus groups convened after the research question and methods have already been determined and operationalized. Such strategic omissions create missed opportunities to make research studies more relevant to the stakeholders working to implement impactful public policy.

A voltage drop diagram (**Fig. 1**) illustrates the potential of academic researchers to influence policy and the relevant factors to consider while attempting to do so. The concept behind a voltage drop diagram is that voltage can be lost in an electrical circuit as current passes through resistors. One of the first uses of a voltage drop diagram in health and health policy depicted the transformation of insurance coverage to quality health care.[27] A voltage drop diagram was also adapted to access and quality in child health services by Chung and Schuster.[28] As shown in **Fig. 1**, our voltage drop diagram displays the many resistors in the circuit between the potential of academic researchers to influence policy and actual policy influence as described above.

Traditional Dissemination of Scientific Information

The traditional model of academic publishing through scientific journals represents another barrier to translating research into policy.[12,13,22] Scholarly content is typically written for scientific audiences rather than general audiences, rendering the work less intellectually accessible to stakeholders external to academic networks. The subscription-based model of academic journals creates another access barrier for general audiences. Even when journals issue press releases to engage larger audiences about specific articles, there may be selection bias toward which articles get featured and failure to highlight findings relevant to policy makers. Publication bias represents another challenge to translating research into policy. This phenomenon, which represents the selective publication of studies based on the direction and magnitude of their findings, leads to studies without statistically significant findings (often termed negative studies) being less likely to be published.[29] Over time, bias is compounded by meta-analysis of results from published studies, leading to overestimation of findings across studies. Publication bias may be particularly harmful if policy makers direct public investments without knowledge of or access to negative studies.

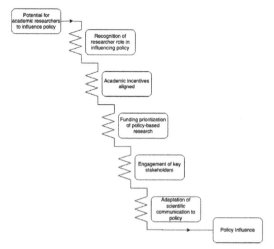

Fig. 1. Potential for academic researchers to influence policy: voltage drop.

Policy Maker Incentives and Approach to Knowledge Translation

Policy makers operate under a different set of incentives than researchers as they are judged by their ability to make impactful change in relatively short political windows. In addition to scientific evidence, policy makers may have other competing influences that drive their decision-making, such as public opinion, professional advocates (ie, lobbyists), and relationships with colleagues.[10,11,30] Attention to constituent priorities and political polling represent a foundational element in decision-making.[31] Professional advocates may influence policy makers through direct lobbying (communication with policy makers) and grassroots lobbying (influencing public opinion to prime voter engagement with policy makers on specific issues).[32] Last, policy makers may be influenced by relationships with their colleagues. Their policy decisions may be impacted by need to align with colleagues or conversely, provide contrast with fellow policy makers. The cumulative consideration of these factors may de-prioritize scientific evidence and create disconnect from translation of research into policy.

Barriers Reflecting the Policy Landscape

In addition to barriers specific to researchers and policy makers, several other factors may influence translation of research to policy.[11,14,30] Researchers and policy makers may encounter substantial obstacles to effective and strategic communication due to different vocabulary and values that may create misalignment of priorities in the policy landscape. The decision-making environment may be impacted by PDOH, limited funding of research by government (eg, gun violence), and budgetary constraints. Last, an immense number of stakeholders may impact child health policy decisions.

EXAMINING THE DISCORDANCE BETWEEN EVIDENCE AND PEDIATRIC HEALTH POLICY

The discordance between the scientific evidence base and policy has been well described and is often attributed to misunderstandings between researchers and research consumers (eg, policy makers), complexities of implementation of evidence into policy, and motivations which may supersede scientific evidence such as bias and structural racism.[15,33] The authors provide three examples based on current topics that demonstrate the discordance that exists between evidence and pediatric health policy.

Child Poverty

In 2016, the American Academy of Pediatrics (AAP) released a policy statement with an overarching synthesis of evidence describing child poverty and recommendations to address child poverty in the United States.[34] The first sentence of the policy statement reads: "Almost half of young children in the United States live in poverty or near poverty." The policy statement further describes opportunities for public policy to mitigate child poverty based on current scientific evidence in **Fig. 2**. Despite these specific policy recommendations synthesizing a strong body of research, there remains a large gap in policies that support children and families in poverty.

As a prime example, home visitation programs for at-risk families have been studied in longitudinal randomized-controlled trials and systematic reviews and reviewed extensively (including by governmental agencies) with multiple efficacious models described.[35] Despite the evidence, these programs remain significantly underfunded presumably due to the perceived long ROI and lower prioritization of social services for underserved populations. The child tax credit enacted during the COVID-19 pandemic represents another missed opportunity to align research to policy. This program was lauded widely in the research community as an evidence-based strategy to lift children and families out of poverty, but has ceased due to a failure of the current congress to structure policy to continue support of the program.[36]

Firearm Injuries

Firearm injuries are annually one of the leading causes of morbidity and mortality among children in the United States. Despite the epidemiology of firearm injuries, the funding to support firearm research and community initiatives to reduce firearm violence is proportionally low even in comparison with other common childhood injuries (such as motor vehicle collisions).[37] It is well-known that the history of firearm policy in the United States is intricate and complex, but several things remain clear according to the evidence when discussing childhood firearm violence:

- Childhood firearm injuries and deaths have risen in the past decade
- Significant racial disparities exist in regard to who is affected by firearm violence
- Middle and high school children are more likely to die from firearm violence than any other cause of death

Despite the existing data, the underlying motivation for policy makers to meaningfully address the issue has been sporadic and fragmented. This is partly because the evidence base is not as robust for firearm violence prevention initiatives in comparison with other childhood injuries due to the Dickey Amendment, which in 1996 inserted the following language into a US federal government omnibus spending bill "none of the funds made available for injury prevention and control at the centers for disease control and prevention (CDC) may be used to advocate or promote gun control." This restriction on federal funding severely limited the firearm research agenda until congress in 2018 clarified the law allowing firearm research, with FY2020 being the first earmarked funds for firearm research since 1996.[38] Legislation such as the Dickey Amendment has made it difficult for researchers to generate evidence and consequently for policy makers to propose and adopt evidence-based programmatic policy.

Motivation of policy makers to address firearm injuries has been undermined by several factors. With strong ties to the firearm industry, the National Rifle Association is one of the well-funded lobbying groups in the United States and has built a legacy of influencing policy makers and voters to restrict policy related to firearms as well as

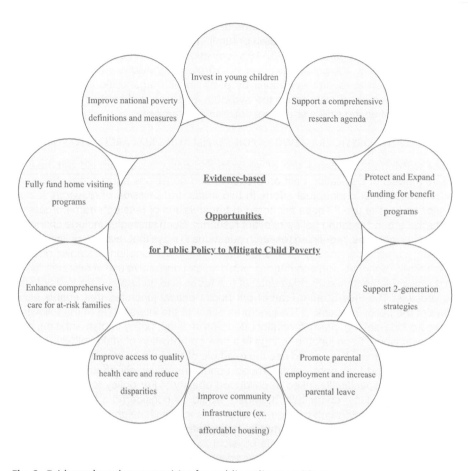

Fig. 2. Evidence-based opportunities for public policy to mitigate.

overtly politicizing the issue. This influence has resulted in inaction on childhood firearm injuries in the United States. Despite these challenges and lack of support, researchers and pediatric professional organizations have persisted in addressing the issue of firearm violence in the United States. The AAP composed of a policy statement of firearm-related injuries in the pediatric population, which similarly to the statement on poverty, suggested multiple policy interventions that could curtail firearm injury based on the available evidence.[39] Many of these policy suggestions are yet to be enacted.

COVID-19 Vaccination

A more recent example of the discordance between evidence and policy derives from COVID19 pandemic and vaccinations. Despite convincing evidence supporting the COVID-19 vaccination of children under 12 years of age in reducing severe disease, public policy has lagged behind, and at times, directly opposed the evidence. It has been postulated that this is due to general mistrust, widespread fear of complications, and poor communication of scientific evidence.[40] As an example, the Florida Department of Public Health announced in March 2022 that it recommended against vaccinating healthy children under the age of 12 citing that the risks outweigh the benefits (https://www.floridahealth.gov/newsroom/2022/03/20220308-FDOH-covid19-vaccination-recommendations-children.pr.html). This recommendation contradicted national guidelines regarding COVID-19 vaccination based on current available evidence (https://www.cdc.gov/vaccines/covid-19/planning/children.html). In this case, the contradiction in recommendations by public health organizations and differing opinions by perceived experts on the available evidence hinders the initiation and continuance of sound policy to protect children and families.

CREATING A THEORETIC FRAMEWORK FOR TRANSLATING RESEARCH INTO POLICY

Those working at the intersection of research and policy have grappled with how to create models of translation built on proactive and conscious approaches. Scholars have focused their conceptual efforts in two areas: *transmission of research* versus *receipt and active use*.[6] Those anchored in transmission of research frame proactive strategies around creating policy-relevant research. Such strategies include changing academic incentives, redefining research questions in ways that relate to policy, active and early stakeholder engagement, and utilization of dissemination strategies outside of academia. Scholars with orientation toward receipt and active use of research focus on policy implementation. Fundamental of this focus is to understand the policy making process. The Five-Stream Framework posits critical junctures that enable each stage of the policy process.[41] The junctures occur at the intersection of the following steps: agenda-setting, policy formation, decision-making, policy implementation, and policy evaluation. Each juncture brings in a new composition of stakeholders, strategies, and resources. If we could use the example of the built environment, it has long been understood that poor neighborhood conditions adversely affect the health of children, more specifically linked to childhood obesity.[42] For policy to be enacted to address this inequity, community members would be considered a key stakeholder for agenda-setting (through their personal experiences with neighborhoods) and policy implementation (notably if community-based interventions such as healthy diet initiatives and methods to increase safe physical activity are undertaken). Researchers could be incorporated at each juncture as an input to advance to the next stage, working directly with other key stakeholders such as community members, media outlets, and policy makers to provide evidence-based strategies to improve the built environment and result in improved health outcomes. For researchers to be successful within this framework, it is crucial to recognize that relationship building represents a cross-cutting construct in all conceptual efforts spanning transmission of research and receipt and active use. Researchers must build strategic partnerships and collaborations with other stakeholders and policy makers.

AN AGENDA TO ADVANCE TRANSLATION OF RESEARCH INTO POLICY

Building on a large body of literature and theoretic frameworks,[4,6,10,14,41,43,44] we outline strategies for researchers to address key gap areas in the promotion of research to policy translation. Themes and strategies to translate research into policy are also summarized in **Table 1**.

Address the Return on Investment Conundrum in Child Health

The long time horizon for ROI of child policy investments necessitates clear articulation to policy makers of how child health differs from adult care and innovative approaches including the use of diverse but meaningful variables, designation of intermediate outcomes, and consideration of outcomes outside of health care (eg, educational attainment, recidivism in the juvenile justice system). The use of outcomes

Table 1	
Themes and strategies to translate research into policy	
Themes	**Strategies**
Address the return on investment (ROI) conundrum in child health	Clear articulation to policy makers of how child health differs from adult care
	Use of diverse but meaningful variables, designation of intermediate outcomes, and consideration of outcomes outside of health care
	Align costs with benefit
	Value-based payment approaches for health care, sharing investments across sectors, estimates of stakeholder-specific returns over policy-relevant timelines, and decreasing silos
Develop a policy-relevant research approach	Modernize: develop research questions, study design, and dissemination with consideration of how scholarship will translate into the policy arena
	"User-oriented" research to provide the data needed by those who can influence policy change
	Learn graphic design, communication science, and the psychology of information processing
	Engage policy makers and relevant change agents where they are and expect and prepare for uncertainty
Prioritize community engagement	Engage multisector stakeholders (outside of the medical center) to establish a win-win situation
	Give voice to community members impacted by the research, notably vulnerable populations
Change the incentives and infrastructure in academic research	Institutions incentivize researchers by including metrics for policy engagement in annual performance evaluations and promotion criteria
	Institutions facilitate relationships with government relations, public relations, and community benefits personnel, legislators, community leaders, philanthropists, and other stakeholders
	Funding agencies: incentivizing researchers to be active in translating research to policy (eg, PCORI)
	Journals increase article types to include policy relevant academic publications and dissemination strategies

in other sectors may exacerbate the wrong pockets problem. Therefore, corresponding strategies that align costs with benefit are needed to address this phenomenon. Strategies to combat the "wrong pockets" problem may include value-based payment approaches for health care, sharing investments across sectors, more detailed estimates of stakeholder specific returns over policy-relevant timelines, and decreasing silos across government agencies.[17]

Develop a Policy-Relevant Research Approach

Researchers must modernize how they develop research questions, study design, and dissemination with consideration of how their scholarship will translate into the policy arena. Furthermore, they must model their work into "user-oriented" research which seeks to provide the data needed by those who can influence policy change.[10] While not a replacement for investigator-initiated research, this approach recognizes the need to tailor the description of findings toward the information priorities of policy makers. Researchers must learn tools such as graphic design, communication science, and the psychology of information processing. Recent work in this area has stressed the importance of disseminating medical and public health research in an accessible manner across electronic platforms, notably social media.[12,13] There are benefits to these strategies, but researchers must recognize the challenges and dangers of this strategy of dissemination as well. **Fig. 3** represents a summary of the benefits, challenges, and strategies to overcome the challenges for use of electronic platforms by researchers aiming to effectively communicate with key stakeholders. Of note, there is overlap in this chart with media-based communications as well, which is another effective strategy for communication of scientific audiences to key stakeholders. In addition, researchers must engage policy makers and relevant change agents where they are.[10] This may include meetings with legislators, agency heads, business executives, and civic officials. Last, researchers must become comfortable navigating the uncertainty in how their work is interpreted or used in the decision-making environment.

Prioritize Community Engagement

Translating research into policy relies on engagement with populations impacted by potential outcomes. This is especially important when engaging traditionally disenfranchised populations, such as racial and ethnic minoritized groups, LGBTQIA+ (Lesbian, Gay, Bisexual, Transgender, Queer/Questioning, Intersex, Asexual, Agender), and individuals with disabilities, who represent populations and communities of individuals who have historically been excluded from research (or directly harmed through medical research) and are frequently the targets of racist and discriminatory public policy. Concrete strategies to help facilitate community engagement include fostering relationships early, well before research project begins; appointing a patient or family member to the research team or a long-term appointment to a research committee or advisory board within the academic institution; and establishing a continued investment in ongoing collaboration, which may not be directly related to research priorities.

Change the Incentives and Infrastructure in Academic Research and Traditional Dissemination

In order for the above strategies to work, there must be corresponding changes in the incentives that underpin academic research. Incentives start with the academic institutions which can make policy and advocacy a core component of their mission and support career development.[22,45–47] Academic institutions can incentivize researchers by including metrics for policy engagement in annual performance evaluations and promotion criteria. To support researcher involvement in policy, institutions can facilitate internal relationships with government relations, public relations, and community benefits personnel and external relationships with legislators, community leaders,

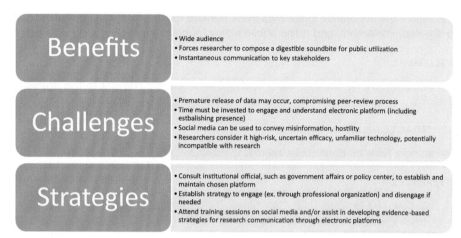

Benefits	• Wide audience • Forces researcher to compose a digestible soundbite for public utilization • Instantaneous communication to key stakeholders
Challenges	• Premature release of data may occur, compromising peer-review process • Time must be invested to engage and understand electronic platform (including estbalishing presence) • Social media can be used to convey misinformation, hostility • Researchers consider it high-risk, uncertain efficacy, unfamiliar technology, potentially incompatible with research
Strategies	• Consult institutional official, such as government affairs or policy center, to establish and maintain chosen platform • Establish strategy to engage (ex. through professional organization) and disengage if needed • Attend training sessions on social media and/or assist in developing evidence-based strategies for research communication through electronic platforms

Fig. 3. Benefits, challenges, and strategies of electronic communication for researchers.

philanthropists, and other stakeholders. Academic institutions can also create internal infrastructure to centralize resources and expertise for pediatric researchers. At certain institutions, these have been labeled policy centers or institutes, with varying goals, foci, personnel, and services (eg, policy research collaborators, policy grants, mentoring, communication, academic-community partnership). Institutions can also support faculty participation in career development programs such as the Health Policy Scholars Program through the Academic Pediatric Association (https://www. academicpeds.org/program/health-policy-scholars-program/) and the Robert Wood Johnson Health Policy Scholars Program. Last, institutions can encourage pediatric research faculty to immerse themselves in government, as consultants to or even employees (on sabbatical, perhaps) within state and federal agencies such as the state Medicaid program or the Federal Department of Health and Human Services to build a cadre of individuals able to translate research to policy within such agencies that have a major impact on children's health.

Funding agencies also play a major role in incentivizing researchers to be active in translating research to policy. Funders such as the Patient-Centered Outcomes Research Institute (PCORI) have already begun to change how research is conceptualized and executed. PCORI has standards for patient-centered outcomes, stakeholder engagement, and dissemination to end users of research. Other funders have adopted similar standards for selected program announcements. Journals have also increased the number of article types they offer to include perspective pieces, policy commentaries, advocacy case studies, and data analyses on policy topics. Last, journals have increasingly leveraged social media to enhance dissemination to key audiences. All of these mechanisms create new incentives for researchers to further invest their efforts toward translating their research into policy.

SUMMARY

With continued need to transform child health toward high-quality care, health equity, and impactful public health programming, research remains a central lever in informing policy creation and implementation. However, several challenges at the level of researchers, policy makers, and the decision-making environment impede research translation. It is imperative to address these barriers to maximize research as an input to develop, implement, and refine public policy for children.

DISCLOSURE

The authors have no commercial or financial relationships relevant to this article to disclose.

POTENTIAL CONFLICT OF INTEREST

The authors have no conflicts of interest to disclose.

REFERENCES

1. Institute of Medicine (US) Committee on Quality of Health Care in America. Crossing the quality chasm: a new health system for the 21st century. Washington, DC: The National Academies Press; 2001.
2. Cartwright N, Hardie J. Evidence-based policy: a practical guide to doing it better. New York: Oxford; 2012.
3. Mirvis DM. From research to public policy: an essential extension of the translation research agenda. Clin Transl Sci 2009;2:379–81.
4. Clancy CM, Glied SA, Lurie N. From research to health policy impact. Health Serv Res 2012;47:337–43.
5. Feder J. Why truth matters: research versus propaganda in the policy debate. Health Serv Res 2003;38:783–7.
6. Davis P, Howden-Chapman P. Translating research findings into health policy. Soc Sci Med 1996;43:865–72.
7. Cheng TL, Bogue CW, Dover GJ. The next 7 Great Achievements in Pediatric Research. Pediatrics 2017;139(5):e20163803.
8. Mishori R. The social determinants of health? time to focus on the political determinants of health. Med Care 2019;57:491–3.
9. Kickbusch I. The political determinants of health–10 years on. BMJ 2015;350:h81.
10. Woolf SH, Purnell JQ, Simon S, et al. Translating research into action: a framework for research that supports advances in population health. Front Public Health Serv Syst Res 2016;5:28–34.
11. Martin K, Mullan Z, Horton R. Overcoming the research to policy gap. Lancet Glob Health 2019;7(Suppl 1):S1–2.
12. Meisel ZF, Gollust SE, Grande D. Translating research for health policy decisions: is it time for researchers to join social media? Acad Med 2016;91:1341–3.
13. Grande D, Gollust SE, Pany M, et al. Translating research for health policy: researchers' perceptions and use of social media. Health Aff 2014;33:1278–85.
14. Emmons KM, Chambers D, Abazeed A. Embracing policy implementation science to ensure translation of evidence to cancer control policy. Transl Behav Med 2021;11:1972–9.
15. Oliver K, Innvar S, Lorenc T, et al. A systematic review of barriers to and facilitators of the use of evidence by policymakers. BMC Health Serv Res 2014;14:2.
16. Currie J. What we say and what we do: why US investments in children's health are falling short. Health Aff 2020;39:1684–92.
17. McCullough JM. Declines in spending despite positive returns on investment: understanding public health's wrong pocket problem. Front Public Health 2019; 7:159.

18. Rees CA, Monuteaux MC, Herdell V, et al. Correlation between National Institutes of Health funding for pediatric research and pediatric disease burden in the US. JAMA Pediatr 2021;175:1236–43.

19. Flores G, Lesley B. Children and U.S. federal policy on health and health care: seen but not heard. JAMA Pediatr 2014;168:1155–63.

20. Caldwell PH, Murphy SB, Butow PN, et al. Clinical trials in children. Lancet 2004; 364:803–11.

21. Groff ML, Offringa M, Emdin A, et al. Publication trends of pediatric and adult randomized controlled trials in general medical journals, 2005-2018: A citation analysis. Children (Basel) 2020;7(12):293.

22. Shah S, Brumberg HL, Kuo A, et al. Academic advocacy and promotion: how to climb a ladder not yet built. J Pediatr 2019;213:4–7 e1.

23. Green LW, Ottoson JM, Garcia C, et al. Diffusion theory and knowledge dissemination, utilization, and integration in public health. Annu Rev Public Health 2009; 30:151–74.

24. Morris ZS, Wooding S, Grant J. The answer is 17 years, what is the question: understanding time lags in translational research. J R Soc Med 2011;104:510–20.

25. Westfall JM, Mold J, Fagnan L. Practice-based research–"Blue Highways" on the NIH roadmap. JAMA 2007;297:403–6.

26. Flynn R, Walton S, Scott SD. Engaging children and families in pediatric Health Research: a scoping review. Res Involv Engagem 2019;5:32.

27. Eisenberg JM, Power EJ. Transforming insurance coverage into quality health care: voltage drops from potential to delivered quality. JAMA 2000;284:2100–7.

28. Chung PJ, Schuster MA. Access and quality in child health services: voltage drops. Health Aff 2004;23:77–87.

29. Joober R, Schmitz N, Annable L, et al. Publication bias: what are the challenges and can they be overcome? J Psychiatry Neurosci 2012;37:149–52.

30. van Schalkwyk MC, Harris M. Translational health policy: towards an integration of academia and policy. J R Soc Med 2018;111:15–7.

31. Blendon RJ, Benson JM. Americans' views on health policy: a fifty-year historical perspective. Health Aff 2001;20:33–46.

32. Landers SH, Sehgal AR. Health care lobbying in the United States. Am J Med 2004;116:474–7.

33. Bailey ZD, Feldman JM, Bassett MT. How structural racism works - racist policies as a root cause of U.S. racial health inequities. N Engl J Med 2021;384:768–73.

34. Council On Community Pediatrics. Poverty and child health in the United States. Pediatrics 2016;137(4):e20160339.

35. Condon EM. Maternal, infant, and early childhood home visiting: a call for a paradigm shift in states' approaches to funding. Policy Polit Nurs Pract 2019;20: 28–40.

36. DeLauro RL. Why we need a permanent expanded and improved child tax credit. Acad Pediatr 2021;21:S90–1.

37. Donnelly KA, Kafashzadeh D, Goyal MK, et al. Barriers to firearm injury research. Am J Prev Med 2020;58:825–31.

38. Rostron A. The Dickey amendment on federal funding for research on gun violence: a legal dissection. Am J Public Health 2018;108:865–7.

39. Dowd MD, Sege RD. Council on Injury, Violence, and Poison Prevention Executive Committee, American Academy of P. Firearm-related injuries affecting the pediatric population. Pediatrics 2012;130:e1416–23.

40. Suran M. Why parents still hesitate to vaccinate their children against COVID-19. JAMA 2022;327:23–5.

41. Howlett M, McConnell A, Perl A. Moving policy theory forward: connecting multiple stream and advocacy coalition frameworks to policy cycle models of analysis. Aust J Public Adm 2016;76:65–79.
42. Singh GK, Siahpush M, Kogan MD. Neighborhood socioeconomic conditions, built environments, and childhood obesity. Health Aff 2010;29:503–12.
43. Woolf SH, Purnell JQ, Simon SM, et al. Translating evidence into population health improvement: strategies and barriers. Annu Rev Public Health 2015;36:463–82.
44. Bernier NF, Clavier C. Public health policy research: making the case for a political science approach. Health Promot Int 2011;26:109–16.
45. Chung RJ, Ramirez MR, Best DL, et al. Advocacy and community engagement: perspectives from pediatric department chairs. J Pediatr 2022;S0022-3476(21): 01224-5.
46. Shah SI, Brumberg HL. Advocating for advocacy in pediatrics: supporting lifelong career trajectories. Pediatrics 2014;134:e1523–7.
47. Nerlinger AL, Shah AN, Beck AF, et al. The Advocacy Portfolio: A Standardized Tool for Documenting Physician Advocacy. Acad Med 2018;93:860–8.

Effective Communication for Child Advocacy

Getting the Message out Beyond Clinic Walls

Perri Klass, MD[a,b,*], Nia Heard-Garris, MD, MSc[c,d], Dipesh Navsaria, MPH, MSLIS, MD[e,f]

KEYWORDS

- Communication • Advocacy • Journalism • Op-ed • Social media • Testimony
- Public speaking

KEY POINTS

- Clinicians can draw on both their direct professional experience and their knowledge of and ability to interpret the research literature to bring a wide audience critical information around many different issues affecting the health and well-being of children, but this kind of communication requires a special set of skills and considerations, which can be taught, practiced, and improved.
- With the ready availability of sometimes dangerous mis- and disinformation and the growth of distrust in traditional authority figures—such as scientists and doctors—this role has become increasingly important for people with medical training, clinical engagement positions, and research experience.
- Clinicians who want to advocate effectively with the general public are advised to think carefully about the messages they most want to deliver effectively, and about the areas where their voices will be most valuable; we then offer specific advice about crafting—and publishing—written advocacy pieces, including op-eds and essays, and about using social media to amplify advocacy.

Continued

[a] Arthur L. Carter Journalism Institute, New York University, 20 Cooper Square, New York NY 10003, USA; [b] Department of Pediatrics, Grossman School of Medicine, New York University, New York, NY, USA; [c] Division of Advanced General Pediatrics and Primary Care, Mary Ann & J. Milburn Smith Child Health Outreach, Research, and Evaluation Center, Ann & Robert H. Lurie Children's Hospital of Chicago, 225 East Chicago Avenue Box #162 Chicago IL 60611, USA; [d] Department of Pediatrics, Northwestern University Feinberg School of Medicine; [e] Department of Pediatrics, University of Wisconsin School of Medicine and Public Health, 600 Highland Avenue H4/4, Madison, WI 53792, USA; [f] Department of Human Development & Family Studies, School of Human Ecology, University of Wisconsin–Madison, 4113 Nancy Nicholas Hall, 1300 Linden Drive, Madison, WI 53706, USA

* Corresponding author. Arthur L. Carter Journalism Institute, New York University, 20 Cooper Square, New York, NY 10003.
E-mail address: perri.klass@nyu.edu

Pediatr Clin N Am 70 (2023) 165–179
https://doi.org/10.1016/j.pcl.2022.09.015
0031-3955/23/© 2022 Elsevier Inc. All rights reserved.

pediatric.theclinics.com

Continued

- Using clinical experiences and anecdotes can offer powerful narratives, but the medical imperatives of confidentiality have to take precedence; we offer suggestions about how to follow journalistic rules of accurate reporting (that is, never make anything up!) while preserving patient privacy and confidentiality.
- Finally, we offer some ideas on public speaking, testifying, and other ways of taking an advocacy message to a larger public.

INTRODUCTION

Effective communication in pediatrics often begins in the examination room, where practitioners discuss many essential—and sometimes fraught—topics with parents and caregivers, beginning with infant sleep and breastfeeding, and continuing, as children grow up, to include conversations with the children themselves, as well as their adults, around vaccination, development, sexuality and gender, mental health, and many more complex and nuanced topics—and beyond that, about any health problems that arise. Many pediatricians take time and thoughtfully consider how to discuss these subjects clearly and helpfully with parents and how to pitch the conversation appropriately for the developmental stage of the child or adolescent. We tend to think of these communication skills as intrinsic to our field; we want people to trust us with some of their most sensitive and private concerns; we want to be nonjudgmental; we want to be clear about the evidence; we want to speak in developmentally and culturally appropriate language—though we may never feel that those examination-room communication skills have been mastered completely.

[Do you see what we're doing here? We're using the first-person plural to draw you in, so that you can identify as part of a larger "we," while establishing that you, the reader, have a certain amount in common with the people writing this piece. We want you to trust us—after all, we have those experiences and emotions in common—while also granting that we may have some special expertise here. We're also trying hard not to use technical terminology, and we are avoiding the passive voice—but on the other hand, we've used the term, "pediatricians," which is often an appealing term to use with the general public—it's clear, specific, with strong positive associations for many people—but having made that point, we should correct that and go on to use a more inclusive term which takes cognizance of the contributions of family physicians, nurse practitioners, and the rest of our valued colleagues.]

In the past, pediatricians—and physicians in general—were generally considered trusted sources of information, and our advice has been highly sought after, but given our current age of information and misinformation overload, the ubiquity of "Dr Google," and a more widespread distrust of health care providers and public health, it is even more important to get these skills right. The era in which physician advice is followed without question is well past us, and no less an authority than the Surgeon General has called misinformation a serious public health threat.[1]

Examination-room communication is vital in clinical practice—but what about when pediatric clinicians want to get some of our most essential messages out to a wider public? How do we take the issues and causes about which we are most passionate and speak from our experience with children and families—clinical, research, public health, professional—in ways that are likely to be effective with a more general audience? This article endeavors to provide some practical guidance to clinicians who want to make that leap to communicating with a wider and less proximal audience.

Let's start from the idea that our clinical experience does in fact give us a valuable perspective from which to contribute to many different kinds of public discourse. But let's also acknowledge frankly that there are some challenges we are likely to encounter as we navigate the complexities of explaining science, of telling stories while honoring patient confidentiality, and perhaps also as we struggle to change our narrative style so that it is less couched in the vocabulary and the conventions of professional medical communication, and more accessible and available to the general reader or listener.

What is Your Message?

The first step, of course, is deciding that there is a conversation that you want to join, a controversy or a discussion about which you feel strongly. This may be a wide-ranging large-scale issue—*vaccines are safe and it's important that children get vaccinated*, for example—or it may be something that has suddenly become a topic of debate in your own community—perhaps something like *youth football and head trauma*, or perhaps some alarm over local toxic exposures, or anything affecting health and well-being. Maybe you've had a clinical encounter that really set you thinking, or maybe a string of clinical encounters have suggested to you that there is a topic very much on the minds of parents in your practice (this is part of how the Flint water crisis came to light through the families in Dr Mona Hanna-Attisha's clinic),[2] or the community in general. Maybe you've found yourself lying awake nights, speechifying inside your head because you're upset—or worried—or angry—or sad. You have something that you want to say, and you think your voice will be valuable.

[Do you see what we're doing here? We're trying to personalize it by switching into the second person—what you are feeling, what you are thinking. We're trying to seduce you into identifying with the narrative—sure, that's me, I've been lying awake, making speeches in my head—I need people to listen to me!]

Where Will Your Voice Be Most Valuable?

This is closely connected to the previous question, but it also considers the sense of obligation and mission that may arise from your special vantage point. Certain topics may go with your particular specialty, with your particular practice, with your own particular experience, perhaps, and not just as a provider, but also as a parent, a patient, or member of a particular community. Any or all of these factors may contribute to your sense of urgency, or your sense of obligation, and give you personal and professional experiences to draw on. It's important to sort this out, because these can also be the experiences, or the qualifications, which you want to highlight in what you write—and they will also help get you the chance to do that writing.

Working on Your Writing Skills

Some of us turn to writing for a more general audience because we have messages we desperately want to get out to the world, but for others, the writing is part of the point—that is, you may want to become a better writer, a more personal writer, a more effective writer. You may be looking for the joy and satisfaction that can come with writing, you may be looking to grow and develop as a writer because you love words and literature. If this is the case, as you consider the question of which issues most engage you, consider as well whether there are ways that you could also develop your writing skills, perhaps by joining a writers' group and exchanging work with other writers, perhaps by taking a workshop or a continuing education course, perhaps by building writing into your daily routine. Writing as a form of advocacy is our focus here, but we want to acknowledge that writing can mean much more than that in our lives (as it does for all three of us) and that there are literary magazines and journals which are specifically interested in voices coming out of health care.[3] You may want to check some of these out, as possible places for your writing, ranging from essays to fiction to poetry.

If you'd like to try approaching editors at some point about advocacy pieces you might write, "marketing" yourself to editors is much easier if you have some "clips," that is, if you can attach or link to other pieces that you've published. And for the most part, scientific journal articles will not really help you here (and neither will poetry); you want to be able to show that you can write effective prose for a general audience. Consider trying an essay for one of the medical journals, which regularly publish such personal pieces, from "In the Moment" in *Academic Pediatrics* to "A Piece of My Mind" in *JAMA*.[4] For many clinicians, these venues can offer a good place to experiment with first-person authorship, and with telling important stories that grow out of clinical and personal experience.

Breaking In/First Steps—the Op-Ed

Okay, you've got an issue that really matters to you (good), and you know what you want to say about it (bravo!). But you have not written for a general audience, and you don't necessarily have contacts in the media. Let's start with the idea that you would like to write an op-ed and place it in your local newspaper. (Shifts in the newspaper industry mean that many may not be reading an actual paper publication, and your piece may only be digitally published—that's fine, but recognize that some of the conventions—and jargon—in what we're about to say come from the days of print-only newspapers.) On the editorial page, the newspaper itself takes positions, in short opinion pieces that are generally unsigned because they reflect the collective editorial opinion, and in this way the paper can comment on current events or weigh in, endorsing candidates. On the contrary, an op-ed is generally a short, signed opinion piece *not* written by someone on the staff of the newspaper, which traditionally runs (in a print newspaper) on the page *op*posite the *ed*itorial page—that's where the term comes from.[5] Writing an op-ed is a perfect way to give your opinion on a specific issue; newspapers are always looking for contributors—and thinking about op-eds is a good way to think about how to lay out an argument.

So let's talk about op-eds

- They tend to have strict word limits—*The Washington Post* gives 750 words as a limit, as does the *Los Angeles Times;* the *Chicago Tribune* says 800, *The New York Times* says 800 to 1200 words. You can search on the Internet for the name of your local paper and "submit op-ed" and you'll get their guidelines, or you can use the information compiled by the OpEd Project.[6] Be sure to check publication websites before submission as their guidelines may change.
- Much helpful information—specific links as well as general advice—is available in the Resources section provided by the OpEd project, cited above.
- Op-eds are generally submitted as full essays, though you can check the website of the newspaper that you want to write for—that is, you don't usually "pitch" an op-ed by writing to the editor to propose the idea (we'll talk about pitching more below); with an op-ed, you generally write the whole piece and submit it through a link on the newspaper's website—something you can do with all of the papers named above and many others.

- Op-eds are designed to be polemical—an op-ed is not the place to hedge or carefully weigh all the different arguments and judiciously allow for the complexities of the discussion; it's a place to make your argument, and you should use every one of those not-so-many words to do that.
- But you should also acknowledge the exceptions, or the most important or weighty objections, with a "to-be-sure" sentence, which, for example, might acknowledge that not every child can be vaccinated, or will respond to vaccines—but you can use that acknowledgment to circle back and emphasize your main point—for example, that vaccinating the vast majority of children who *can* be vaccinated and *do* respond protects the others as well.
- Op-eds are designed to be timely—ideally there is a "peg" or a "hook" which ties your piece to something which has just been covered in the news—in many cases, your chances of seeing the op-ed published will be greater if it comes in right away, while the original news story is still fresh in people's minds. In theory, for many editors, an op-ed is written in the white heat of passion—anger—outrage—concern—celebration—responding to something that has been in the paper in the very recent past.
- When you start writing an op-ed, you need to establish right away both what that argument is, and who you are in the context of that argument—that is, why your opinion should count.
- Think about how to sum that up in a couple of short sentences—you will notice that nowadays, many op-eds run with headlines that essentially say, *I'm this, do that*; one of us wrote a column which ran with the headline, "I'm a Pediatrician. Get Your Child Vaccinated." (The author's proposed title, which she continues to prefer, was "If you were my kid, you'd be vaccinated).") Be aware that authors do not get to determine the title, the pull quote—the short excerpt which sometimes appears in larger type—or the illustration in most cases, though we will suggest below that you ask at least to see all these in advance in case any inaccuracies arise. **Box 1**
- Make it clear in the first paragraph what it is that you are advocating, but do it, if possible, by means of an anecdote that establishes your authority in this area—maybe the story of a patient you saw (see below for a discussion of consent and confidentiality), or something a parent said to you—and then, having used this to establish why this issue is on your mind, lay out what you are advocating as clearly and unequivocally as possible.
- Then build your case—a little history if necessary, a little science, another personal anecdote if you have one.
- If you are writing for a local paper, make this as local as you can: In my practice in the such-and-such neighborhood, a problem they're seeing at the such-and-such food pantry, a controversy which has come up at the such-and-such school. You want them to see you as an expert, but also as someone who knows

---

Box 1
Advocacy Anecdotes

I once wrote about the need for universal health care (this was back in the Clinton administration) by beginning (first sentence) with a story of a child I had seen in clinic the night the President made his health care speech—the child needed an oral antibiotic for a skin infection but had no health coverage; the mother did not have the $23 so the health center paid—the point of this example was that it was so "humdrum," so every day; *not* a life-threatening emergency but a universal feature of daily practice, needing a universal solution.

the territory and is a part of the community. Language that signals your familiarity, that shows you know, for example, which are the important parks, the important hometown sports teams, the beloved local snacks, will help with this.

- Do not use anybody else's language—organizations sometimes provide "talking points" or "boiler plate" but you should use this only to check your own work, to make sure you've covered all the major issues. We live in an era when it is very easy to go on the Internet and find out if something is original, or if the same language has been used elsewhere. You are going to sign this piece, so make sure the words are your own. If someone says something in a particularly pithy or memorable way, you can quote it—but as a general rule, don't quote press releases or publicists.
- Think about how you may want to reference your personal experience, perhaps your identity, perhaps your family experiences—stories and anecdotes make anything easier to read, but in an op-ed they really have to serve the central argument (we'll discuss issues of privacy and confidentiality below).
- End on an emphatic call-to-arms restatement of your argument—speak with urgency, say what needs to happen and why.
- Ask a colleague whose writing (and thinking) you respect to look it over and let you know if anything is ambiguous, unclear, or problematic—this is especially important if you are new to this kind of writing. Consider asking a colleague whose views actually differ from your own to tell you whether you have used language which will offend or polarize; you want people who don't agree with you to read what you've written (or what's the point?). **Box 2**
- And then go ahead and upload it, following the newspaper's directions.
- Op-eds are meant to be timely, so you should hear back within a couple of days. Generally, you can only submit to one news outlet at a time—the website may tell you that they do not allow simultaneous submissions. You can emphasize this by saying in an accompanying email that you are offering this piece as an exclusive to the paper, but will need to offer it elsewhere if you do not hear back within 3 to 4 days. And indeed, if you do not hear back—and especially if the issue is indeed one where you have tied your piece to something in the news, feel free to send a nudging email asking whether they think they will be able to use your op-ed. And then, having nudged, feel free to submit it on another newspaper's website (if suddenly both places want it, well, you'll cross that bridge when you come to it—or, as one of our grandmothers might have said, that should be your biggest problem!). You can consider your follow-up query a notification that if they don't respond, you need to move on.

What About Doing All This on Social Media?

Social media and self-publish platforms, like *Medium* and others, offer both opportunities and challenges—the opportunity is the easy potential reach to such a large

---

Box 2
Advocacy Anecdotes

A colleague—with the best of intentions—took me up on an offer to review a draft op-ed and offer advice and suggestions. Despite some guidelines being offered, the draft was about three times longer than the newspaper's limits, was filled with journal citations, and much of it was fairly technical. When these issues were gently pointed out, the author stated his coauthors wanted it to be even longer. The diplomatic response was that a piece that needed this much work was unlikely to even get a response from an editor.

audience, the lack of an editor-as-gatekeeper, and is generally less-formal nature. It's a challenge for all the same reasons, of course. Good editors (and we hope they are all good) can help reshape writing, can serve as a check on something that perhaps should not go out, and can prevent overly-casual communications when the topic deserves gravitas and carefully chosen words.

The journalist A.J. Liebling once wrote, "Freedom of the press is guaranteed only to those who own one;"[7] social media effectively gives every user a "press." However, a distribution network doesn't automatically come with your new social media "press." Sure, the technical framework is there, but without networks of followers, or adroit use of tags, your well-crafted message may not go anywhere. Alternatively, in obedience to Murphy's Law, your clumsy joke or the snarky comment you immediately regretted may go viral.

So, the same basic advice that we went over above regarding op-eds generally holds in terms of the content of what you write on social media; you need to craft your message responsibly and effectively while protecting patient privacy and yourself. If you're new to this—or even if you're not—a good strategy may again be to ask a colleague whose judgment you trust to glance at your advocacy-related social media posts before you hit "send," just to cross-check, to make sure that you've got the tone right, and to double check that you didn't miss anything.

Social media can amplify your non-online advocacy work as well. Commonly, when visiting legislative staff during a "Hill Day", we'll ask for a photo with the staffer, which is almost always a "yes." (Even in an era of online "Hill visits," a screenshot of the Zoom room—again, with permission—works well.) Soon after the visit, post it with a thank you to the staffer (by name—they almost never get public thanks!), and tagging the elected official's account is valuable. Why? Not only are you thanking them, you're publicly announcing why you were there. It reminds them that you're not only an individual, or a small group of people meeting with them, but you also reach an awful lot of other people, including…yes, other, constituents.

Each social media platform makes use of "tags" in different ways, and therefore we won't even attempt to go through each one. While tagging matters, what makes the most difference is your online reputation, which is what will draw people to follow you and then to spread your material to their own networks. So, work to curate that online reputation with care, using your real name and professional credentials. Always write accurately and responsibly, but stay away from jargon and endless technical information. Pass along material only from other people you trust—if you're new to a platform, you would do well to spend a few months simply "listening" to what others say to gain a sense of the culture and who's involved.

And finally, remember that your social media persona is not separate from who you are as a person—how you behave on social media reflects on you in reality. That can be negative—name-calling, flame wars, and other "bad behavior" can paint a rather unseemly picture of you that can spill over into the in-person world. But it can also be positive—how you are on social media can benefit the "you" that shows up to speak at conferences, as a professional colleague, or as a clinician…and vice versa. Although social media's "hierarchy of needs" may at its base be about safety and security (don't share patient info, don't embarrass yourself, etc.), at its peak it is about innovation and discovering new ways to improve human health, including advocacy work.[9]

Going Beyond the op-Ed: How to Pitch Longer Articles and Essays

You may wish to write a longer article or essay. The approach tends to be somewhat different: as we said above, op-eds are generally submitted in full. An editor may approach you with an idea, but generally, these opinion editors are not particularly receptive to being "pitched." Op-eds are short, and many of the websites with guidelines specify that they are only interested in seeing complete pieces. However, if you want to write a longer piece, a more analytical (and less polemical) piece, a piece that will not necessarily run on that proverbial page opposite the editorials, you may well find yourself in the position of writing a pitch: *here's a piece I want to write, here's why you should want me to write it.* It's basically a proposal for what you'd like to write.

In general, you will find that you are much more likely to be able to get the tone of your articles and op-eds right if you are writing for publications that you actually read, and this will also be true of the pitch. Thus, it's a good idea to personalize your pitch a little, making it clear that you know and respect the publication, explaining why this particular story is right for this particular publication: *because it is so well trusted in our community, because it is such a great source of information for parents, because it has such a strong record of investigative reporting and advocacy…*

The pitch itself should simply be an email to the relevant editor (most publications make email addresses for specific editors or for general pitches available on their mastheads) which should do the following:

- Explain what the piece is that you want to write. Remember that you will be judged for your writing ability by the person reading the email, so it should be lucid, grammatically flawless, and generally representative of your writing voice (which is, it goes without saying, lucid, and grammatically flawless).
- Tell them who your audience is—is this directed at parents who are trying to navigate a confusing or potentially scary medical territory, or is this directed at the general public who will understand an important public health issue better—and make sure that your language and your writing are in keeping.
- Explain why you are the right person to write it. This gives you a chance to write a paragraph about who you are and what you do and why you care about this issue.
- Offer the names of the media outlets and links to any other pieces you have published.

[Do you see what we're doing here? We're addressing the reader directly, offering specific guidance in short bites—as you might in a "service piece," that is, an article aimed at helping parents figure out what is best for their children. The sentences are short, and the language is decidedly nontechnical; for example, we didn't use the term "service piece" in one of the bullets.]

The sad truth, as most writers know, is that pitch letters don't always get answered. There is no rule that says you can't send the same pitch letter to multiple editors, though it's always worth taking the trouble to touch it up a little so that it's tuned to each new publication. Nobody likes reading form letters.

Writing for a Wide Audience—Telling Your Stories Effectively

What you most *don't* want to do—and what editors may be most afraid that you will do—is write this in a way that is too academic. We sometimes become accustomed, in medicine, to the diction and vocabulary which are routinely used to communicate important information, with all appropriate precision, caution, and (let's face it) jargon. There's nothing wrong with using technical language to communicate technical information to a group of people all grounded in the field, but editors, depending on the experiences that they have had with people writing from within medicine, may be profoundly wary of us, expecting language that will frankly lose the nonspecialized reader. Doctors, in particular, have something of a reputation as bad communicators (back in the pre-computer days, jokes about illegible handwriting were a staple), and although we may feel that things are generally brighter in pediatrics, there are plenty of locutions which sound normal to us, and still come off as specialized or technical.

Here's the most important single piece of advice (and it gets more important the more academic writing you've done): avoid the passive voice. Don't use it. Take to heart what Strunk and White say as their 14th principle of composition in *The Elements of Style:* "The active voice is usually more direct and vigorous."[8]

[Do you see what we're doing here? We didn't say, the passive voice is to be avoided, whenever possible. It is not to be used.]

Have a really low threshold for explaining your terminology, if you do have to use specialized words, and explain them without reference to other specialized words. Don't assume people know what a NICU is (even if you write it out), don't assume people know what a live-virus vaccine is, don't assume people know the difference between anesthesia and analgesia, or between prophylaxis and treatment (actually, people may well known all those things—but editors are often worried that they won't, or that they'll be discouraged by too many science words).

Using Stories from Your Clinical Practice: the Confidentiality Imperative

Do use stories and anecdotes from your clinical practice, and as far as possible, personalize them by identifying the general area where you practice so your readers know that you are referencing children in your community. You are a clinician, and this experience is your superpower. Using this superpower immediately brings up the issue of patient confidentiality, of course, a complex topic for any of us who write about medicine, and one which does not easily lend itself to simple rules. Our first responsibility, it should go without saying (but let's say it anyway), is to our patients, and we can't allow that confidentiality to be endangered in any way. Medical journals allow you to change names and details, but the rules are different in journalism; you can leave out information (no one has to know that this issue came up because the child was in your examination room with his brand-new twin sisters) but you can't make anything up.

So how do you navigate confidentiality and the divergent ethical priorities of medicine and journalism? If there's a really compelling story you want to tell, and you think that it's going to be recognizable to the patient and family (and even more if it's going to be recognizable to other people), your only option is to ask permission, explaining that you won't use any names or identifying details. And even if the family gives you permission, there may well be stories you don't feel right about using. All of us who write about medicine carry around a certain backlog of stories which just can't be told because they aren't ours, or it wouldn't be right because there's no way to tell them without identifying details. And on the other hand, there are families who have wanted their stories told—even families who have asked to have their names used. **Box 3**.

Box 3
Advocacy Anecdotes

I once wrote an essay about taking care of a child who had received a liver transplant, and referred to the child only by her initial. Because the case was so distinct and recognizable (not so many liver transplants in your average primary care practice), I showed the essay to the parents before publication, and their only request was to change the initial to the real—and unusual—first name of the child; the parents had become activists for pediatric organ donation, and pointed out that the child's medical story—with her name—was already posted on transplant advocacy sites, and they wanted to be sure that people knew the story was about her.

If you change identifying details, you need to specify that in your writing, either by saying that you've changed the details or by saying something like, "I will call him John, which is not his real name, and let's say he was 5, which is not his actual age." But by the rules of journalism, that means that you have not, for example, made Jane into John, or made your stressed-out junior varsity hockey star into a stressed-out varsity football player. Some editors at some publications may be okay with the I-will-call-him-John approach, others may not; there are many places where if you say, "I will call her D.," then D has to be the real first letter of her name.

Alternatively, you can choose a story which is pretty generic, or write about it in a way which makes it clear that you are combining stories: "I seem to be having the same conversation over and over with parents about vaccination—I say such-and-such—they say such-and-such—one father said such-and-such—one adolescent said such-and-such." That lets you pack in a number of quotes without giving any identifying details about different patients.

You can dwell in more detail on your own thoughts and emotions, as you are not walled off from those by any confidentiality concerns, and also because those may be most interesting to your audience. You are letting them in on your feelings as a clinician, using the patient stories as prompts. You can also use stories from your own family (though even there it's important to get consent; you don't want your middle-school kid to find out that you've been telling stories out of school by hearing about it *in* school. **Box 4**.

Avoiding Academic Diction

We often want to write about studies and science—and bringing science to bear on decision making can be a really important part of advocacy, whether that's individual decision-making (get your kid vaccinated!) or policy level advocacy (get everybody vaccinated!). Be particularly aware of the complexities of research words—significant (or not significant), study limitations, control group. Explain what you're saying, explain why you're citing a particular study, explain what kind of study it was—you can't just say, pilot, or observational, or longitudinal double-blind controlled. And be patient and precise about explaining the difference between correlation and causation, which trips up many editors (that is, the experience of writing about scientific studies may involve carefully explaining why a study shows an interesting correlation (say, spicy food and longer life expectancy) but cannot be read as indicating a causal relationship, and then, after all that, you may find yourself looking at a headline that says, "Eating Hot Peppers Makes You Live Longer!") And though, as we said above, the writer does not generally get to write the headline, you should by all means ask the editor to run the headline, the illustration, and the caption by you—for the sake of medical accuracy. **Box 5**.

Getting Blowback: Controversy and Criticism

There are journalists who measure the success of their polemics by the anger and hostility they arouse. It's an honorable tradition within the field of journalism, but it's not generally what clinicians are looking for when we spill over into writing for the general

---

Box 4
Advocacy Anecdotes

When I wrote an essay about my preschool-aged son, even though he was much too young to give consent, the journal required I get signed consent/permission from his dad.

> **Box 5**
> **Advocacy Anecdotes**
>
> I write a regular column in a local newspaper, and the editor chose a lovely, cute photograph of a baby sound asleep, illustrating the preciousness of life, which connected somewhat to the themes of the written piece. Unfortunately, the baby was asleep on its stomach, on rather soft bedding. When shared on social media, a fellow pediatrician didn't comment at all on the column, but criticized the photo for depicting unsafe sleep practices. From then on, I have asked to be able to review photo choices, just to avoid inadvertent pediatric no-nos.

public. In an era in which many public health interventions have become sadly politicized, putting yourself out there in the popular press, or on social media, can sometimes mean encountering hostility and, in extreme cases, even being publicly attacked or having your practice targeted, for example, with negative online reviews. If this happens to you, consider contacting your institutional public affairs office, or your local AAP chapter (or, in the event of threats, law enforcement agencies) and requesting advice.

Commenting for the Media

When it comes to advocacy, speaking up and speaking out in the newspapers, on TV, on social media, can lead to more opportunities—and specifically to the chance to quite literally do some speaking. It's another reason to choose your issues carefully; if you've started to write about something that's in the news, people will start to see you as someone who can be called on for expertise, and you may well find yourself invited to comment—and be quoted—in news stories, to speak at meetings, to be part of panels, or to give testimony in the political process. You want to spend your time and energy on the issues that matter to you.

Let's start with the question of giving comments to journalists, which means putting yourself and your opinions out there, and let's be clear, you may not be offered the chance to do the kind of editing and revising and considering that you were able to do on your own piece. If the outlet or the publication or the show is unfamiliar to you, do your research—find out the reputation of the host who will be interviewing you, find out if the show has a strong political bent. Most journalists will be conscientious, reasonably prepared, reasonably unbiased—but there are occasionally hostile situations and you don't want to be taken by surprise. If your institution has a media relations office, they may be able to help you prepare.

If you've been asked to comment on a particularly controversial issue for an article someone else is writing—you're now an expert, after all—and you're worried about getting the language exactly right, you can ask the journalist, can I email you a few comments. You can also ask whether any quotes that are going to be used can be checked with you, either read back to you or emailed to you—though you generally cannot ask to see the whole article. This is because it's actually not considered good journalism practice to run your article past your sources, but it is *very* good practice to double-check your information, so ask to check your quotes to make sure that you've been clear and accurate—which is, in fact, exactly what you want to be.

If you're giving a spoken comment, on TV or radio, get to your point directly. In fact, if you have a main point you want to make about the issue, you need to make that point pretty much regardless of what question you are asked. If you know you'll need more time than you're going to get (most TV comments are quite short), consider linking to social media and elaborating there. But your actual comment should emphasize whatever is your most important point, and if you have a little more time, you might want to repeat it. If you get asked a question which seems off topic, or which you don't particularly want to answer, don't refuse to answer (or, worse, say "no comment"), but instead use a technique called "bridging:" find a way to get back to the point you want to make, which can be as blunt as saying, "I think the really important issue here is...." And stick to your point; the old adage about telling your audience what you're going to say, saying it, and telling them you've just told them really applies to giving comments; you're in this game to get your message across. **Box 6**.

The person who is interviewing you may be a generalist who knows just a little about the topic, or may have reported on it in depth and know a great deal — you should try to get a sense of this at the beginning of the interview — before the tape is running. Someone who really knows the subject can help you get a sense of how to use your time most effectively, and it's fine to ask that question. Remember that your comments will also be edited; you may find that your 20-minute interview ends up being more like 20 seconds, especially if it's for television. Or you may find yourself faced with a live interview, usually lasting only a couple of minutes, in which your strongest imperative, again, will be to hit your most important message as hard as you can — regardless of what you are asked. Radio sometimes gives you more time, and public radio in particular.

What about Public Speaking and Testimony?

Your reputation is growing — now you're being asked to be on a panel, to speak at a meeting, to testify at the state capitol. All of these represent real opportunities to get your message out, maybe to bring about important change.

Testifying

Here is where you often will prepare a written statement, complete with facts and figures, which you will put into the official record, and you may well hand out copies. Treat it as you would an op-ed; make your key points as clearly and forcefully as possible, and if the hearing concerns a particular policy or bill, say exactly what you think should happen. Use your personal voice, your anecdotes, your local connections. If you have access to a government affairs office, you should seek out their help with this and understand the political landscape to offer a more effective testimony. Also, don't forget to call yourself "Doctor" — this is not the time to be a typically self-effacing, modest pediatrician! **Box 7**.

If possible, get to the hearing early, and listen to what other people say in testimony. There may be questions you want to clear up, or comments you want to respond to — you can add some ad libs into your testimony. **Box 8**.

Choose your stats carefully; go for studies which do not take too much explaining. It's important — again — to avoid jargon, so you need a study you can explain without too many annotations. You need to be accurate, but you do not need to follow

---

Box 6
Advocacy Anecdotes

I was in clinic when a candidate for governor arrived for a visit, with reporters in tow. After a brief conversation with the candidate in the hallway, a reporter approached me and asked, among other things, who I supported in the election. I wasn't going to say that at all, but particularly not while standing in clinic while displaying my work ID. I simply replied "Children's health shouldn't be a partisan issue. I am happy to work with anyone who cares about improving the lives of children and families." They asked a second time, and I gave the same answer. They gave up after that—I didn't get "trapped," and I kept the focus on the issue.

> **Box 7**
> **Advocacy Anecdotes**
>
> I was asked to testify in a State Senate committee alongside the Senator introducing a bill we supported. It became clear that they wanted to show they had "the pediatric society" on their side. Of course, I did this when I was 'just' an intern, but it didn't matter—I was an MD, and I was there on behalf of our State AAP Chapter.

scientific-journal standards of pointing out all limitations; the qualifiers that lend weight in scientific discourse can create all kinds of issues and misunderstandings. Your job here is to frame the study so that it makes sense for a general audience, so that they understand the take-home point, and hear that point made by a trusted voice—yours.

Speechifying

Let's start by agreeing that spoken advocacy and written advocacy involve different styles, different approaches, different locutions—in other words, do not read your written work! In fact, much as we all love reading aloud (the authors of this article know each other through Reach Out and Read), we need to tell you that public speaking should *never* involve reading prepared remarks. Speak from notes, speak from the heart, but do not read.

Think about your setting—pay careful attention to your time limitations—and think about whether you want to do this with visuals—that is, usually, with slides. The slides, for the most part, should really be *visuals,* not word slides, but if there is a particularly sticky complex statement you want to make, where you will have to pick your words really carefully, you can put that on a slide for emphasis and read that one slide aloud (but the emphasis will be lost if you've shown a lot of word slides and read them all). Slides are there to support your talk—they are not the entirety of your talk.

- Connect with your audience—know who they are, respect them, acknowledge their expertise, acknowledge that you may be telling them things they already know

> **Box 8**
> **Advocacy Anecdotes**
>
> I once testified at a state legislative hearing in support of a bill that would require any youth athlete suspected of having a head injury that may result in a concussion to be removed from play until cleared to return by a professional with expertise in the management of concussion. The most effective messenger was not any of the sports medicine physicians or pediatricians in the room. It was the former star high school quarterback who played on despite a concussion, suffered second impact syndrome, and the ensuing damage meant that he—now in just his 20s—required a cane and his mother's help to walk up to the table to testify. It brought home the dangers in a way that no statistics, study, or even anecdote ever could.
>
> Having said that, carefully listening to prior testimony—and questions—can help. One legislator had a concern that the bill's provisions would be so restrictive that it would essentially prevent youth sports from ever occurring. He asked a question of a health care professional who was testifying, who didn't quite understand the concern. It was clear that the legislator was not in favor of the bill, simply by looking at his face and hearing the tone in his voice. When I testified, after finishing the prepared testimony, I went on to comment on a question that had come up earlier, and offered my own interpretation of what I believe it meant. The legislator in question did not say a word but nodded, appeared satisfied, and went on to vote in favor of the bill.

- Let your passion and emotion come through—remember why you started with this issue, why it matters to you, why you want people to care, what you want to accomplish.
- But don't just tell them why this is important to *you;* tell them how it connects to what they care about—tell them if you're here to help them with issues that are frustrating them, to answer their questions **Box 9**
- Definitely practice your remarks, and consider practicing them on a friend who doesn't work in health care and will be alert for things you might need to explain more fully
- If you know someone who is good at this, ask for honest feedback—ask if there are pieces of your talk which aren't clear, or aren't quite working
- Time yourself! Don't kid yourself about time; the world is full of people who think they've spoken for about 10 minutes when they've really talked for 20—we are all susceptible to the magical sound of our own voices. Don't rely on the venue to have a clock where you can see it—bring your own, or set up your computer to show you the time elapsed. Far better than being only halfway through your talk when someone holds up the "5 min remaining" sign!
- Make 'em laugh. Make 'em cry. The most successful speeches do both—and they do both because you've connected with your audience, they can see that you care—and they understand why

Parting Thoughts

Those who choose to go into health care are often driven by a strong sense of mission. Many of us, let's face it, are also driven by personal urgencies which tend to make us conscientious, driven, self-critical, and even prone to perfectionism, imposter syndrome, and self-doubt, and medical training certainly tends to turn up the volume on all that. Writing for that wider audience, speaking to that wider audience, can sometimes feel like venturing outside that professional comfort zone (where the passive voice is so well appreciated), but the skills and the passion and the energy that drive your clinical work, that urge you into the arena of advocacy, will truly stand you in very good stead as you master these new skills, which will draw in so many ways on the skills you already possess.

Humans are story-telling and story-loving animals. Our clinical work lets us into many, many stories, and gives us the chance—we hope—to shape those stories, to help children and families toward better outcomes and more hopeful trajectories, one examination room at a time. Advocacy offers us a way to use our

---

Box 9
Advocacy Anecdotes

I was at a local pediatric clinic to do a training for Reach Out and Read, which this clinic was soon to implement. A physician walked in, grousing to his colleagues about having to be at this meeting, saying that he couldn't even get into the online training system, and being rather negative about the whole thing. One of our staff did help him with resetting his password, but the biggest success came from the presentation, which focuses on child and family well-being, empathizes with how challenging educational and socio-emotional problems are for clinicians to address, particularly as children grow older, and only then offers ROR as a practical, workable approach for prevention within the context of the existing well-child visit. The same physician who came in annoyed and disengaged came right up at the end and asked when the books were arriving, because he couldn't wait to start participating. It was a remarkable example of how helping people solve the problems they have works so much better than simply trying to "sell your thing," as worthy as it might be.

experiences—and our stories—on a larger scale, to fix up the world or improve the odds for people who may never step into our examination rooms. The world needs your voice, and the stories that you have to tell.

[Do you see what we're doing here? We're offering a peroration, a final wrap-up which uses language from our opening paragraphs and also, that's a little more high-faluting, to remind you that with clinical work—and with advocacy—we have both privilege and opportunity—in other words, we're trying to make you laugh and make you cry.]

DISCLOSURE

All three authors state that they have no commercial or financial conflicts of interest. Drs Heard-Garris, Klass, and Navsaria serve on the ROR National Board, in Board member, National Medical Director, and Board Chair capacities, respectively, all uncompensated.

REFERENCES

1. Murthy VH. Confronting health misinformation: The U.S. Surgeon General's advisory on building a health information environment. 2021. https://www.hhs.gov/sites/default/files/surgeon-general-misinformation-advisory.pdf. Accessed October 21, 2022.
2. Bock E. Pediatrician who uncovered Flint water crisis recounts experience. NIH Rec 2021;LXXIII. Available at: https://nihrecord.nih.gov/2021/04/30/pediatrician-who-uncovered-flint-water-crisis-recounts-experience. Accessed October 21, 2022.
3. Stanford Center for Biomedical Ethics, Medicine & the Muse Program. Places to submit your work. https://med.stanford.edu/medicineandthemuse/ProgramLinks/Journals.html. Accessed October 21, 2022.
4. Florida State University Maguire Medical Library. Publish your work: medical narratives. 2022. https://med-fsu.libguides.com/publishing/narratives. Accessed October 21, 2022.
5. Kennedy School Communications Program Harvard. How to write an op-ed or column. https://projects.iq.harvard.edu/files/hks-communications-program/files/new_seglin_how_to_write_an_oped_1_25_17_7.pdf. Accessed October 21, 2022.
6. The OpEd Project. Submission Information. https://www.theopedproject.org/submissions. Accessed October 21, 2022.
7. Liebling AJ. The wayward press: do you belong in journalism? New Yorker 1960;(May 4):105–12.
8. Strunk W, White EB. The Elements of style. Fourth Edition. New York: Pearson; 2000. p. 18–9.
9. Chretien KC, Kind T. Climbing social media in medicine's hierarchy of needs. Acad Med 2014;89(10):1318–20.

Going Farther by Going Together
Collaboration as a Tool in Advocacy

Shetal Shah, MD, FAAP

KEYWORDS

- Advocacy • Pediatrics • Child health policy

KEY POINTS

- Advocacy is a key element of pediatric care targeting social determinants of health.
- Pediatricians can advance their policy objectives on behalf of children by collaborating with key organizations/partners as part of a coalition.
- For a coalition to be successful, specific objectives, roles, and responsibilities must be established before beginning work.
- Potential collaborating organizations based on age and advocacy issues are provided to facilitate coalition-building.

INTRODUCTION

Over the past two decades, greater attention has been paid to the social influences that impact child health outcomes. Factors such as poverty, health care access, parental stability, food insecurity, and the physical environment are consistently associated with decreased educational attainment, child mental health, shortened life expectancy, obesity, and child substance use.[1–7] Overall, social circumstances contribute ~15% to premature death.[8] With this awareness has come more focus on advocacy in support of remedies that mitigate the adverse social conditions children face. In this context, issues such as expanding universal pre-kindergarten education, child health insurance coverage, housing policies that promote environmental justice and the child tax credit can be considered health care policies.[9] The Centers for Disease Control and Prevention now recognizes social determinants of health as a health indicator and has incorporated them into Healthy People 2030 targets.[10,11] Further the Accreditation Committee on Graduate Medical Education requires pediatric trainees to be exposed to and understand social drivers of health and develop advocacy skills.[12,13]

Division of Newborn Medicine C-225A, Department of Pediatrics, Maria Fareri Children's Hospital, New York Medical College, 100 Woods Road, Valhalla, NY 10595, USA
E-mail address: Shahs2@wcmc.com

Pediatr Clin N Am 70 (2023) 181–191
https://doi.org/10.1016/j.pcl.2022.09.007
0031-3955/23/© 2022 Elsevier Inc. All rights reserved.

DEFINING ADVOCACY

Child health advocacy has multiple definitions, but is based on the intentions of those who founded pediatric medicine. The most encompassing definition describes advocacy as a physician's actions that mitigate threats to health, specifically detailing work that seeks social, economic, educational, or political change conducted under the banner of a doctor's professional work.[14] As distinct from actions on behalf of an individual patient, child health advocacy broadly includes work not restricted to clinical venues.[15] This work has been embedded in medical practice for over 175 years. Writing in 1848, Virchow noted, "Physicians surely are the natural advocates of the poor and the social problem falls within their scope."[16] Almost half a century later, at the dawn of modern pediatrics as a specialty, Abraham Jacobi stated, "[The Pediatrician] is the legitimate advisor to the judge and jury, and a seat for the physician in the councils of the republic is what the people have the right to demand."[16] At the founding of the American Academy of Pediatrics (AAP), Issac Abt noted pediatricians should not just "discover neglected problems," but "correct evils and introduce reforms."[17] Simply stated, advocacy is where the system fails and requires political redress.[18,19]

In an era when threats to short and long-term child health result from their early exposure to adverse social, physical, emotional, and economic circumstances, legislative advocacy has matured to be an essential tool for influencing child well-being. A critical element of legislative advocacy is coalition building. Coalitions enhance advocacy efforts by coordinating resources and multiplying outreach efforts, thereby increasing the odds of success for a shared goal. Further, coalitions have greater credibility than "lone wolf" advocates or single organizations. This is especially important for issues related to children, where individual organizations are often under-resourced or have expertise in one domain (in our case, the health aspect) of any child-related issue.

EXAMPLES OF SUCCESSFUL COALITIONS

Across the spectrum of child advocacy, multiple instances exist of effective coalitions, which can be as small as a few departments in a large medical center or include hundreds of local, state, and national groups representing various constituencies. For example, Jarvis and colleagues,[20] seeking to expand perinatal screening for depression, convened a task force including the primary care division, emergency department, social work, and the neonatal intensive care unit at a major children's hospital—all of whom were aware of the problem within their silo, but unaware of the work done by others. Attempting to reduce youth vaping rates by prohibiting the sale of flavored tobacco products in a county of 1.3 million, New York Chapter 2 of the AAP convened a group of stakeholders including pediatricians, middle- and high-school age children, parent–teacher association (PTA) representatives, legislators, local hospitals, other physician groups and local chapters of the Campaign for Tobacco-Free Kids, American Heart Association, American Lung Association, and American Cancer Society.[21] At the state level, pediatricians and public health researchers worked to reduce infant mortality in Indiana by recruiting state infant mortality review commission members, early childhood education providers, community liaisons, the state department of corrections, and a documentary film crew to create a grass-roots system of leaders to promote maternal-child health in communities with high infant mortality.[22] Finally, Quinlan and colleagues,[23] working nationally, partnered with the federal Consumer Product Safety Commission, Underwriter's Laboratories, and a children's product safety organization called "Kids in Danger," to create a new standard to make microwave oven doors child-resistant. As acknowledged by these authors, none of the projects would have succeeded without assistance from their assembled coalition.

PRACTICAL STEPS IN COALITION BUILDING

Building a coalition to further an advocacy goal is straightforward, but requires attention to the roles, benefits, and assets each member brings toward the achievement of the stated goal. In general, coalitions expand inversely to time commitment (**Fig. 1**). That is, the less resources/time you ask another organization to provide and the less work you ask them to do, the more likely they will join the coalition, but also the more discerning you should be about their specific contribution. Forming a successful coalition requires several key elements[24]:

1. As the group is formed, it is essential for defined roles to be assigned for each group. This allows for more effective and productive work, reducing duplication of effort and assumptions that others are performing a task.
2. The process of decision-making must be clearly articulated from the outset. When the coalition disagrees, how is a decision made? By the "heavy lifters" most involved? Majority rule? Etc.
3. The contributions, benefit, and value for each group should be defined. What can each group realistically commit in terms of human resources, networks, and economic assets?
4. Periodic reassessment of roles and resources assigned to the project by each member should occur. Advocacy is a marathon, not a sprint—even "simple" goals can take longer to achieve and, particularly for advocacy, multiple legislative sessions. What a coalition member can provide over the time frame may be different at mile 20 than it was a mile 1.

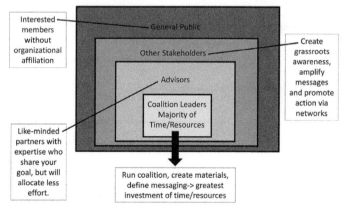

Anatomy of a Coalition

Fig. 1. A schematic representing potential roles for organizations/individuals who are members of a coalition. Leaders will shoulder the greatest burden of work associated with the issue, but defining roles and resources from other coalition members is integral to overall success. (*Adapted from* reference 24. Community Catalyst. Roadmaps to Health Community Grants Advocacy Toolkit. Coalition Building and Maintenance. Available at: https://www.communitycatalyst.org/resources/tools/roadmaps-to-health/coalition-building-and-maintenance (Accessed May 24, 2022).

Fortunately, because pediatricians are relatively respected and children are often the focus of organizations, there exist many potential community groups eager to partner. See **Fig. 2** for an excerpted list of child-focused organizations restricted to a certain age groups. An exhaustive list can be found at the Community Pediatrics Training Initiative.[25,26] Coalitions related to a specific issue can be seen in **Table 1**.

EXAMPLES OF COALITION BUILDING

An example of the strength and unexpected benefits of a strong, well-organized coalition can be seen in an AAP chapter-based advocacy project to prohibit the sale of flavored nicotine products. Partnering with a local county legislator in a suburban community of New York City, the coalition contained multiple associations dedicated to reducing the impact of tobacco on youth.[21] These included organizations such as the American Heart Association, Lung Association, and Cancer Society, as well as local PTA groups, superintendents, the American College of Chest Physicians and Parents Against Vaping and E-cigarettes (PAVE). Though this coalition grew and ultimately included individual parents, students, local hospitals and school districts, the initial group assigned clear tasks and responsibilities to each member based on available resources. AAP, for example, would provide educational briefings to legislators, conduct in-person meetings with lawmakers, and help craft the bill to be inclusive of available tobacco products. PAVE would speak in favor of the bill at assigned committee hearings, author letters of support and activate their large member listserv encouraging members to call their county representatives ahead of key votes to demonstrate grassroots support. Other organizations provided testimony at committee meetings and provided technical assistance and data included in the legislative presentations AAP conducted. The elected legislators and staff guided the process of creating and moving legislation, arranged for briefings with colleagues, coordinated media outreach, and convened press conferences.[21] By defining roles at the onset of the project, the coalition

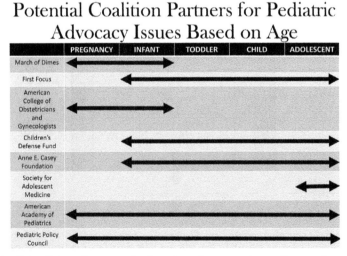

Potential Coalition Partners for Pediatric Advocacy Issues Based on Age

Fig. 2. Potential collaborating organizations based on age. Across the spectrum of pediatrics, stakeholders often focus on specific age ranges. As you build your coalition, consider partnering with organizations that focus on your intended age range. Note that several of these organizations are dedicated to child-related issues, but are not composed of physicians, which expands the support your issue may receive.

Table 1
Sample advocacy partners by subject/policy focus

Issue	Organization
Nicotine/tobacco control	• Campaign for Tobacco-Free Kids • American Heart Association • American Lung Association • American Cancer Society • American College of Chest Physicians • Parents Against Vaping and Electronic Cigarettes • Local Health Departments
Medicaid	• State American Academy of Pediatrics Chapter • Georgetown Center for Children and Families • Campaign for Better Health Care • Doctors for America • Physicians for a National Healthcare System • Local Health Departments • State Medicaid Office
Injury prevention	• Safe Kids Worldwide • Child Injury Prevention Alliance • Prevention Institute • Children's Safety Network • Local Health Departments
Mental health	• National Alliance on Mental Illness • American Psychiatric Association • Mental Health America • American Academy of Child and Adolescent Psychiatry • Local Health Departments
Gun violence	• Everytown for Gun Safety • Brady Foundation • Moms Demand Action
Food insecurity	• Feeding America Action • Food Research and Action Center • State Anti-Hunger Organizations • Local Food Banks

Multiple organizations may serve as potential collaborators and coalition members on advocacy issues of interest to pediatricians. List are an excerpted list of partner organizations pediatricians may consider allying with based on the specific issue of concern.

prevented in-fighting, made clear delegated responsibilities, and was able to pivot after several votes in support of the measure failed. After this setback, the networks and additional skills within the coalition allowed for a rapid change in tactics, moving to pass similar bills in the towns which comprise the county. For example, our legislator's staff decided what town boards would be most receptive to rapidly passing this proposal. PAVE and AAP members who lived in these towns were contacted and local PTA members were recruited through the informal networks of these groups (friends, business associates, and friend-of-a-friend) These community members assisted with scheduling PTA-supported information sessions at local schools located in these town before votes. At the town level, having 10 to 20 advocates in support of child-friendly legislation was uncommon, and allowed for unanimous passage of a prohibition on the sale of flavored nicotine in several towns. Once a large number of local towns passed the measure, county approval was inevitable.[21]

The above case demonstrates the importance and value of partnering with your local AAP chapter to assist and support advocacy efforts. It also highlights the need to tailor your coalition to the region or constituencies In this case, local PTA members, pediatricians, and parents residing in the towns proved more influential than larger national and physician-led organizations, which may have been viewed as too distant or removed from these local political issues. These stakeholders, however, would not be appropriate for potential national legislation. Consider the efforts from the Society for Pediatric Research to support the Research Investment to Spark the Economy Act—which would provide supplemental funding and timeframes for scientific grants to provide flexibility due to COVID-19-related issues.[27] Local coalitions would be of limited value for this national issue, and partners would better include groups with a national perspective, such as the Federation of Societies for Experimental Biology, or existing coalitions that have local organizations as members, such as the Ad Hoc Group for Medical Research, as well as Congressional offices from districts which receive substantial federal extramural research support.

LOCAL AMERICAN ACADEMY OF PEDIATRICS CHAPTER

Aside from organizations outlined in **Table 1** and **Fig. 2**. Other groups exist with missions compatible with the most common pediatric advocacy issues. These partners should assist advocates in refining and researching their topic, and can form the basis of your coalition, most prominentl among these is the local AAP Chapter. As the local chapter operates most closely to pediatrics in your region, basic information about their structures, mission, and membership is worth reviewing. The National AAP works closely with independent local chapters, which maintain separate membership distinct from the national organization. Currently, 59 US-Based and 7 Canadian Chapters comprise the organization. With the exception of California and New York State, each state, as well as Puerto Rico and Washington DC hosts a chapter.[28] In partnership with the National Committee on State Government Affairs, local chapters are a natural home to begin building your coalition. Most chapters have reliable, existing partnerships with local child-friendly advocacy groups, established relationships with state legislators and regulatory officials, and often ties to local academic pediatric programs in the state. For example, New Jersey pediatric residency programs created a joint advocacy collaborative with support from the state AAP Chapter. The chapter leveraged existing local relationships to recruit faculty for a "Virtual House Call" series of webinars.[29] For legislative advocacy local chapters almost universally have advocacy staff or contracts for legislative services, which can expand the reach and influence of any proposed legislative work. Further, most chapters host annual "Advocacy Days" where pediatricians visit the state capital and meet directly with legislative staff to promote bills of interest. Having your issue included on these agendas is another means of expanding an issue's footprint and gaining coalition support.[30] Chapters may also have strong relationships with the state Medicaid office and local county, city, and state departments of health, which can provide another expert voice on the potential impact of proposed health regulations. However, as local government agencies, these groups may be less inclined to vocally advocate for either specific regulation or legislation. Finally, local issue-specific groups, such as local chapters of Moms Demand Action or Everytown for Gun Safety for concerns about firearm safety or Mothers against Drunk Driving for impaired driving and injury prevention may also be beneficial.

NATIONAL ORGANIZATIONS

National organizations also can assist in joining or building coalitions for suitable issues that are federal in scope. The Pediatric Policy Council, which advances policy goals mutually agreed upon by four national-member organizations: the Association of Medical School Pediatric Department Chairs, the Academic Pediatric Association, the American Pediatric Society, and the Society for Pediatric Research—promotes issues related to academic pediatrics. Currently, this includes a focus on the development of the pediatric scientist pipeline, subspecialty loan repayment, federal support for the educational mission of children's hospitals, funding for the National Institutes of Health, and Medicaid remedies that increase access to care. In addition, member organizations maintain separate advocacy committees to work on affiliated projects.

The Academic Pediatric Association has created a Health Policy Scholars Program, a 3-year mentored partnership to help build and execute an advocacy project while simultaneously creating academic work products to assist in promotion. The program combines formal education in coalition building and a structured program to advance your specific priority. The National AAP participates in multiple coalitions to advance its agenda-most notably during 2017 efforts to repeal the Affordable Care Act—legislation which increased the number of insured children via Medicaid Expansion and creation of health care insurance exchanges. In the spring of that year, the American Health Care Act passed the House of Representatives, marking the first major legislative threat to the Affordable Care Act since its creation in 2010. The bill would have reduced Medicaid spending, eliminated the individual and employer mandate to purchase health insurance, eliminated tax credits to offset the price of health care, reduced essential health benefits, and changes the rules allowing insurance premium differences for those with pre-existing conditions.[31] Multiple Senate versions of the repeal, including the Better Care Reconciliation Act, which phased out Medicaid Expansion, the Health Care Freedom Act, which repealed the Affordable Care Act without replacement provisions, and the Cassidy-Graham bill to provide block grants to states to fund health care all failed.[32] Pushing against such strong forces required a fellowship of 6 major physician groups, causing AAP to field a coalition that included the American College of Obstetricians and Gynecologists (ACOG), the American Osteopathic Association, the American Academy of Family Physicians, the American College of Physicians and the American Psychiatric Association.[33] This group represented ~500,000 US physicians, and staunchly opposed the repeal of the Affordable Care Act. As repeal efforts failed, this group provided a loud physician voice against removing key elements of the law.[34]

Several other nonmedical nation organizations have large child-health/welfare portfolios. For example, First Focus on Children is a large bipartisan advocacy organization aimed at ensuring children are fairly represented in federal policy and budget decision-making. UNICEF provides support for children internationally, focusing on international vaccine delivery, water quality and sanitation, maternal/child health, and nutrition. The Children's Defense Fund is another large non-partisan nonprofit organization dedicated to serving the needs of children, particularly those in poverty or from under-represented groups. The organization focuses on preventive physical and mental health care but works at both the federal and state level.

ROLE OF A NATIONAL ORGANIZATION FOR A LOCAL ISSUE

Even if an issue is state-based or regional, national organizations can provide expertise not available locally. The AAP Section on Neonatal-Perinatal Medicine has worked to assist neonatologists seeking state-based Medicaid coverage for pasteurized human donor milk, obtained primarily from non-profit human milk banks, as a means to potentially reduce the incidence of necrotizing enterocolitis. The group recruited interested neonatologists in states without Medicaid coverage and provided a toolkit with a sample letter of support, template legislation, and a spreadsheet to assist on cost estimates if potential legislation targeted very low birthweight infants.[35] The group provided each neonatologist with seed funding, required partnership with the local AAP Chapter, and advised coalition building, which included Regional Perinatal Centers, ACOG, Midwifery groups, safety-net hospitals, and mothers of infants with necrotizing enterocolitis. By providing this assistance, the section buoyed efforts leading to the passage of bills in Georgia, Washington State, Ohio, and Florida.[36] Though the national organization did not elevate this to federal policy, it created important linkages to neonatal experts in advocacy, donor milk, and necrotizing enterocolitis to assist on-the-ground efforts in states, advising on coalition building and AAP Chapter partnerships.

NATIONAL RESOLUTIONS

National AAP assistance is based upon your advocacy work being consistent with published policy statements issued by the academy. However, not all child-friendly ideas are represented in AAP policy. To increase the visibility of your issue before creating a coalition and providing input on an organizational agenda, engaging with their policy and proposal process may be necessary. Work with the AAP is again instructive, as the academy's infrastructure provides a formal mechanism by which to potentially direct policy via the resolution process. Annually the academic solicits resolutions from members which instruct potential new policies. Resolutions require support from a chapter, section, council or committee of the academy and are debated at an annual leadership conference, where they are formally adopted or rejected. Attendees at the leadership forum rank the Top 10 resolutions which go directly to the national board of directors. Resolutions can have a profound impact on state-based advocacy. The neonatal section's work on Medicaid coverage for donor milk began as a resolution. Similarly, resolutions supporting in-hospital vaccination of new mothers against influenza and pertussis formed the basis for the 2009 Neonatal Influenza Protection Act and the 2012 Neonatal Pertussis Prevention Act. Resolutions in 2015 calling for AAP to terminate sponsorship on its HealthChildren. org website by companies that produce soft drinks and sugar-sweetened beverages resulted in the academy removing Coca-Cola as a sponsor.[37] Hence resolutions remain another avenue to expand your advocacy reach and ultimately recruit coalition members.

SUMMARY

Coalition-building is a critical skill and part of any successful advocacy strategy. Creating a successful coalition follows a pattern that includes:

1. Defining your advocacy goal.
2. If your goal is not part of an organization's agenda, consider the resolution process or similar mechanism to place it there.
3. Recruit coalition members that supplement your knowledge-based or provide additional resources and perspectives to the goal.
4. Plan and assign roles based on the time/resources each coalition member can allocate. Include a process for decision-making if opinions differ.
5. Amplify your goal by working with local state or federal agencies to provide expertise and guidance.
   . 6Meet with coalition members often to assess progress, re-evaluate workload, and recruit/engage new partners.

Multiple local, state, and federal partners exist to include in your coalition and should be tailored to your audience and advocacy outcome. Finally, multiple examples of successful coalitions in pediatric advocacy exist upon which to base your work.

CLINICS CARE POINTS

- Coalitions are an essential element of child health advocacy, distributing workload, enhancing impact, and broadening the scope of your work.
- Successful coalitions involve organizations with shared objectives, but different and mutually beneficial skills.
- To optimize collaboration, roles for different organizations must be defined beforehand and periodically revaluated.

DISCLOSURE

The authors have nothing to disclose.

REFERENCES

1. Allensworth DD. Addressing the social determinants of health of children and youth: a role for SOPHE members. Health Educ Behav 2011 Aug;38(4):331–8.
2. Campbell F, Conti G, Heckman JJ, et al. Early Childhood Investments Substantially Boost Adult Health. Science 2014;343(6178):1478–85.
3. Metallinos-Katsaras E, Must A, Gorman K. A Longitudinal Study of Food Insecurity on Obesity in Preschool Children. J Acad Nutr Diet 2012;112(12):1949–58.
4. Zimmer KP, Minkovitz CS. Maternal depression: an old problem that merits increased recognition by child health care practitioners. Curr Opin Pediatr 2003;15(6):636–40.
5. Levinson M, Parvez B, Aboudi DA, et al. Impact of Maternal Stressors and Neonatal Clinical Factors on Post-Partum Depression Screening Scores. J Matern Fetal Neonatal Med 2022;35(7):1328–36.
6. Wood DL, Valdez B, Hayashi T, et al. Health of Homeless Children and Housed, Poor Children. Pediatrics 1990;86(6):858–66.
7. Aysola J, Orav EJ, Ayanian JZ. Neighborhood Characteristics Associated With Access To Patient-Centered Medical Homes For Children. Health Aff 2011; 30(11):2080–9.
8. McGinnis JM, Williams-Russo P, Knickman JR. The case for more active policy attention to health promotion. Health Aff (Millwood) 2002 Mar-Apr;21(2):78–93.
9. Palfrey JS, Tonniges TF, Green M, et al. Introduction: Addressing the millennial morbidity–the context of community pediatrics. Pediatrics 2005 Apr;115(4 Suppl):1121–3.
10. Centers for Disease Control and Prevention. Social Determinants of Health (SDOH): Know What Affects Health. Available at: https://www.cdc.gov/socialdeterminants/about.html. Accessed 5 May 26, 2022.
11. U.S. Department of Health and Human Services. Office of Disease Prevention and Health Promotion. Healthy People 2030. Social Determinants Health. Available at: https://health.gov/healthypeople/priority-areas/social-determinants-health. Accessed May 26, 2022.
12. Rezet B, Risko W, Blaschke GS, et al. Dyson Community Pediatrics Training Initiative Curriculum Committee. Competency in community pediatrics: consensus

statement of the Dyson Initiative Curriculum Committee. Pediatrics 2005;115(4): 1172–83.

13. Marsh MC, Supples S, McLaurin-Jiang S, et al. Introducing the concepts of advocacy and social determinants of health within the pediatric clerkship. MedEdPORTAL 2019;15:10798.

14. Earnest MA, Wong SL, Federico SG. Perspective: Physician advocacy: what is it and how do we do it? Acad Med 2010 Jan;85(1):63–7.

15. Christoffel KK. Public health advocacy: Process and product. Am J Public Health 2000;90:722–6.

16. Virchow R. Collected essays of public health and epidemiology. Cambridge, England: Science History Pubns; 1985.

17. The American Academy of Pediatrics. 90 Years of caring for children 1930-2020. American Academy of Pediatrics 90th Anniversary Publication; 2020. Available at: https://downloads.aap.org/AAP/PDF/9.%20AAP%2090TH%20ANNIVERSARY% 20-%20FINAL.pdf. Accessed May 27, 2022.

18. Rudolph MC, Bundle A, Damman A, et al: Exploring the scope for advocacy by paediatricians. Arch Dis Child 1999;81:515-518.

19. Paulson JA. Pediatric Advocacy. Pediatr Clin North Am 2001;48(5):1307–18.

20. Jarvis L, Long M, Theodorou P, et al. Perinatal Mental Health Task Force: Integrating Care Across a Pediatric Hospital Setting. Pediatrics 2021 Dec 1;148(6). e2021050300.

21. Shah S, Siddiqui S, Meltzer Krief E. Advocacy Case Study: Restricting the Sale of Electronic Nicotine Delivery System Flavors. Pediatrics 2021;148(3). e2021051223.

22. Turman JE Jr, Swigonski NL. Changing Systems That Influence Birth Outcomes in Marginalized Zip Codes. Pediatrics 2021;148(1). e2020049651.

23. Quinlan KP, Lowell G, Robinson M, et al. Making Microwave Oven Doors Child Resistant to Protect Young Children From Severe Scalds. Pediatrics 2021; 147(2). e2020021519.

24. Community Catalyst. Roadmaps to Health Community Grants Advocacy Toolkit. Coalition Building and Maintenance. Available at: https://www. communitycatalyst.org/resources/tools/roadmaps-to-health/coalition-building-and-maintenance. Accessed May 24, 2022.

25. Hoffman BD, Rose J, Best D, et al. The Community Pediatrics Training Initiative Project Planning Tool: A Practical Approach to Community-Based Advocacy. MedEdPORTAL 2017;13:10630.

26. American Academy of Pediatrics, Community Pediatrics Training Initiative. Project Planning Tool: Developing a Community Advocacy Project Proposal. Available at: https://www.aap.org/en/advocacy/community-health-and-advocacy/ community-pediatrics-training-initiatives/. Accessed March 10, 2022.

27. House Resolution 869. Research Investment to Spark the Economy Act of 2021. Available at: https://www.congress.gov/bill/117th-congress/house-bill/869/text? r=2&s=1. Accessed May 26, 2022.

28. American Academy of Pediatrics. Community. District Map. Available at: https:// www.aap.org/en/community/district-map/. Accessed May 26, 2022.

29. Traba C, Pai S, Bode S, et al. Building a Community Partnership in a Pandemic: NJ Pediatric Residency Advocacy Collaborative. Pediatrics 2021;147(4). e2020012252.

30. Chapter Advocacy Days Lay Groundwork for Legislative Wins. American Academy of Pediatrics, AAP NEWS June 23, 2017. Available at: https://publications. aap.org/aapnews/news/8226. Accessed May 27, 2022.

31. House Resolution 1628. American Health Care Act of 2017. Available at: https://www.congress.gov/bill/115th-congress/house-bill/1628/text. Accessed May 28, 2022.

32. Cohn J. The ten year war: obamacare and the unfinished crusade for universal coverage. New York: Martin's Press; 2021.

33. Joint Recommendations of the American Academy of Family Physicians, American Academy of Pediatrics, American Congress of Obstetricians and Gynecologists, American College of Physicians, American Osteopathic Association, and American Psychiatric Association on Priorities for Coverage, Benefits and Consumer Protections Changes, April 11, 2017. Available at: https://osteopathic.org/2017/04/11/medical-groups-including-aoa-issue-joint-recommendations-for-health-care-reform/. Accessed March 10, 2022.

34. Affordable Care Act Repeal without Replacement Harms Patients. America's frontline physicians reiterate opposition to any effort that leaves patients worse off. American Academy of Pediatrics, American Academy of Family Physicians, American College of Physicians, American College of Obstetricians and Gynecologists, American Osteopathic Association, American Psychiatric Association; 2017. Available at: https://www.aafp.org/dam/AAFP/documents/advocacy/coverage/aca/LT-Group6-SenateACA-Repeal-071917.pdf. Accessed March 10, 2022.

35. Schmaltz CH, Bouchet-Horwitz J, Summers L. Advocating for pasteurized donor human milk: the journey for medicaid reimbursement in New York State. Adv Neonatal Care 2019;19:431–40.

36. Shah S, Miller ER. Advocating for Donor Milk Access in Medicaid: Bringing Equity to the Neonatal Intensive Care Unit. Pediatr Res. Available at: https://www.nature.com/articles/s41390-021-01807-w.pdf. Accessed May 28, 2022.

37. Woodruff J, Sreenivasan H, O'Connor A. American Academy of Pediatrics decides relationship with Coke is not so sweet. 9/30/15. Available at: https://www.pbs.org/newshour/show/coke. Accessed May 25, 22.

Moving?

Make sure your subscription moves with you!

To notify us of your new address, find your **Clinics Account Number** (located on your mailing label above your name), and contact customer service at:

Email: journalscustomerservice-usa@elsevier.com

800-654-2452 (subscribers in the U.S. & Canada)
314-447-8871 (subscribers outside of the U.S. & Canada)

Fax number: 314-447-8029

Elsevier Health Sciences Division
Subscription Customer Service
3251 Riverport Lane
Maryland Heights, MO 63043

*To ensure uninterrupted delivery of your subscription, please notify us at least 4 weeks in advance of move.

Printed and bound by CPI Group (UK) Ltd, Croydon, CR0 4YY

03/10/2024

01040467-0002